PARENTING TODDLERS

The best guide complete with tips and tricks on how to discipline toddlers and Adhd kids. Grow your children consciously without giving up the playful side of parenting.

SOFIA WILSON

Table of Contents

BOOK 1: TODDLERS DISCIPLINE

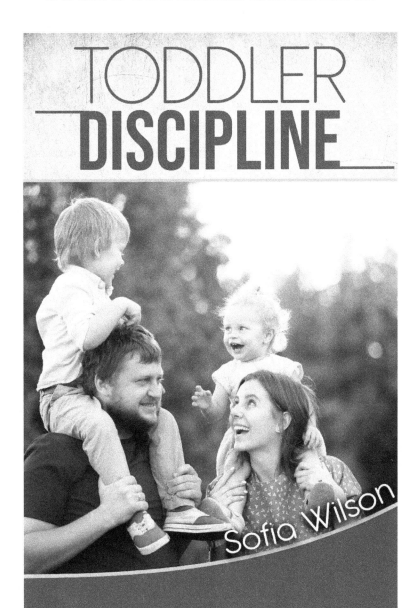

Introduction

While you can see the physical growth that your toddler experiences as they age, you cannot see their minds working. The brain of a toddler is also under constant development, as your little one learns more about the world around them. This includes learning about the things that they can achieve, what they are physically capable of, as well as exploring their boundaries and growing into their independence. It is around this age that they first start to explore life without their parents or their primary caretaker. To establish this independence, it is important that your child has room to explore the way they want to. However, he or she also must be corrected and given boundaries.

Before you jump into disciplining and correcting your child for their misbehavior, it is important to deeply study what is going on in their minds. While you cannot let your child do whatever they want, you must also show empathy for their thought processes and all the emotions they are experiencing for the first time. This will create a deeper connection between you and your child. It will also build the type of relationship that helps you discipline, while still remaining supportive and understanding.

The toddler age is generally used to refer to children one to two years old, referring to the toddling they do as they learn to walk. It is a time of physical and emotional development. Your little one is learning to explore all the ways they can interact with the world around them. They are also learning what is expected of them. It is important to remember that being a toddler should be a learning process for your child. They are learning what they are allowed to do. They are learning where they fit into the world and falling into a role. With the right nurturing, this role they fall into will guide them, as they grow into a productive, respectful, well-behaved members of society.

Common Toddler Behaviors

In the first few years of their children's lives, most parents find themselves wondering if how their child is behaving is normal. There are not that many behaviors that are unusual for toddlers.

Temper Tantrums: Toddlers throw temper tantrums for several reasons. Sometimes, they are hungry or tired, and that causes irrational responses to the world around them.

Irrational Crying: Toddlers will cry about anything, from losing their favorite blanket to their sandwich being cut the wrong way. When your little one seems like they are being irrational, they are likely experiencing some emotions they are unfamiliar with. Having an environment that is too overstimulating can also cause irrational crying.

Problems Sharing: Generally, kids are taught that it is good to share with their friends. At the toddler ages, however, kids are more likely to want to play by themselves or next to another child, rather than playing directly with them. While socialization is important, do not be surprised when your little one does not want to share their favorite toy. Additionally, while you should encourage your son or daughter to share, it is also important that they learn to respect others' belongings. You can do this by encouraging others to respect the toddler's belongings as well.

Difficulty Paying Attention: You cannot lecture a toddler because they lose interest after the first sentence. You should also expect them to switch tasks frequently throughout the day, as many things will not hold their attention for very long.

Saying No: Every parent dreads that moment when their toddler says no for the first time. It is often the first time many as toddlers learn to assert their independence and dominance in the world. Saying no should be expected—you will learn how to handle it.

Hitting, Biting, Scratching, etc.: Playing with friends is not always cute. Toddlers lack the social skills to express their emotions and may react undesirably by hitting, biting, scratching, and screaming when they do not get their way. You will learn more about how to handle these undesirable behaviors in the right way.

Why Toddlers Do Not Listen

Toddlers do not spend every minute of the day being obedient. While this desire to get something immediately lies at the root of many listening problems, there are other reasons your toddler may not listen as well, including the following:

They are imitating you: Toddlers are sponges, soaking up everything from the world around them. They also look to their parents and caretakers for guidance. That means if their caretaker is doing something, even if the child is not allowed to do it, they may mimic the behavior. This applies to all behaviors—even things like interrupting, not listening to others, talking loudly, or fighting with your spouse. Give your toddler the same listening and respect that you would expect them to give you or another adult.

They are bored: Toddlers have a short attention span. If what you are making them do is less enjoyable than what they would rather be doing, it may be a struggle getting your little one to listen.

You lectured: Lecturing a toddler does not yield results. Rather, toddlers will become glass-eyed after the first few words of your sentence.

You are using the wrong words: Word choice is important when you are speaking to a toddler. They have a natural aversion to words like no, cannot, and do not. Rather than using words like *not hitting* or *not running*, put a positive spin on it: make short, affirmative rules like, "We are kind to others," or "We walk in the house."

There is no follow through: If you are constantly repeating yourself and your child continues not to listen, without consequence, they will not take you seriously. It is important that consequences are put into place and used when your toddler makes the decision not to follow a rule. You can increase effectiveness by being consistent with consequences.

You yell: Some parents resort to yelling at their toddler. While this could be useful in dangerous situations, using a loud tone loses its effectiveness when it is done all the time. It teaches your child that when you are loud, you mean business, and they do not have to listen otherwise.

They were not listening: Children can be very involved with whatever their mind is focused on at the time. It is critical that you have their attention before you tell them what you want them to do. Otherwise, you will find that you must repeat yourself.

Turning off the electronics or removing whatever is distracting them at the time can also be helpful.

Your child feels out of control: Not all children are focused on the aspect of control in their lives since some are more independent than others. If you have a child that wants to exercise their independence, you should let them. Give them a way to feel in control, even while getting them to do what you want. You will learn how to create this illusion of control.

Of course, this only covers some of the reasons that toddlers do not listen. Like mentioned earlier, sometimes there is no underlying cause—they would just rather do what they are doing than listen to you.

Chapter 1:Improving Your Toddler's Behavior

Communication with your child represents an open door. The child will often initiate a conversation (sometimes it can be an open invitation for help), but the question is whether you will recognize this call for help, hear it, and answer it with an adequate response. If you invest in communicating with your child, this communication becomes the foundation on which you will build a lasting relationship.

Some of the basic laws of good communication with your child are

1. Consider their age. You can already begin to explain the great secrets of life to your three-year-old child. It is surprising, but your toddler can understand how children are born, whether there is a God, what happens when someone dies, and similar things. Still, when you are talking to a child, the principle is always the same: tell the truth, using words the child is already familiar with. Communication is a two-way street when you share your everyday experiences with a child, rather than expecting them just to talk to you. If you get a detailed answer to the question of how your toddler spent the day, the child deserves to receive a detailed answer to his question as well.

2. Share your personal opinions. You do not have to always keep things in confidence just because of the different levels of a child's thinking. It is your duty to always state your opinion, that is, what you believe to be right, but in

a manner that does not hurt your child, does not diminish him or her, or underestimate him. Just talk.

3. Always show your child enough patience and time to talk. If your toddler grows up with the conviction that he can communicate with his parents, he will feel safer and happier. Try setting priorities. If your toddler wants to talk to you, while you are doing some housework, let your child do so.

Communication is learned. Occasional quarrels, conflicts, and misunderstandings are common and typical occurrences in communication: never give up.

Speech is given to us, but the art of conversation is learned. We all can hear, but to understand, we have to put effort, time, and love into learning to listen.

How to control the child's aggression:

From time to time, your child will get bruises and scratches, not only from taking a fall, but also from playing games with their friends. Children have always played "mother and daughter" and "catch." It might seem like you could just say to your child: "Give the doll to Katie, you are a good girl!" But even if your child does it, you may not know what feelings are at work inside her. Maybe she will get the impression that it might not feel so good to be good.

If you see or suspect how difficult it is for a two-year-old child to part with their favorite toy, for the sake of good manners, it is better not to push the child and not to bring on hysterics.

When your toddler becomes a little older and has more experience in communicating, as much as possible, to try to predict them.

Often, parents are worried about situations in which their child might be aggressive, taking a toy from another child. Almost all kids struggle if they are somewhat dissatisfied and behave badly if they are tired. Sometimes the aggressiveness of the child results in your toddler biting other children. This is basically the same situation.

If a quarrel does not lead to outright aggression on the part of one or more of the children, parents should not interfere. If there is a need to intervene, do not try to name a culprit: for one of the children, your decision will still be unfair.

It is better to intervene on the quarrel and divert their attention to other activities. If you see that one of the children is constantly antagonizing your child, look for another circle of friendship, at least for some time, where the relationship between children will be somewhat different.

If you observe a situation in which your two-year-old child is hitting other children, do not spank them or physically discipline them in any way, and, of course, do not ask another child to do it.

Perhaps your toddler is too small to respect other children. This respect needs to be learned gradually. Take the child aside, and at the same time, explain that they hurt the other child, and that your child needs to apologize to him or her. If there is an opportunity, let your bully play with older children: in that type of environment, it will be harder for them to try to prove their strength. Note: the older the child, the more selective your toddler will be regarding demonstrations of his own aggressiveness towards other people. Most likely, children are aware of what they can get away with it and what they cannot.

In any case, children should be taught systematically to share toys

If your child reveals an aggressiveness that frightens you, you need to think perhaps, of its origins: for instance, the relationships that have developed in your family. Do not forget that you are an example to your child. And yet, the skills of exhibiting a good attitude towards each other are better instilled when the child is in good humor.

Outpouring Of Feelings

Teach your toddler to be concerned about everyone around them. Let them help you while cooking: put the dishes on the table with you, put out bread and fruit. And you should accompany their actions with encouraging words. It will take more time to complete the task than if the child wasn't "helping you," but you have learned that feeding a child is not all there is to raising him or her. Remember this.

You might put a doll or a toy animal down to sleep, gently stroking them "before bed," saying that they have been good and obedient. Ask your toddler to show how he or she loves the doll or toy animal.

Show your toddler how to take care of flowers, paying attention to the fact that they have beautiful small delicate leaves and flowers.

When you go for a walk, take food for birds or squirrels in the park, feed them together, and praise the toddler for it.

If the child is sad or overexcited, then perhaps he will not do what you ask of them. Perhaps they will break a leaf, throw the doll on the floor, or will not want to feed the animals.

This temporary act of aggression does not indicate bad character traits at all.

A sense of parental love and tenderness gives a child the opportunity to feel good and gives him or her confidence in life.

What Is Good and What Is Bad

While a baby is small, the main prohibitions given by the parents are related to the concern for his or her safety. Always, when forbidding something and saying the word no, do not forget to explain why and to tell the child how or what he needs to do instead. In addition, parents should know that praise is much more instructive than limitations.

As often as possible, show approval for the good things your toddler does, especially those that were hard for them to complete. Do not simply give them prohibitions. According to psychologists, verbal restraints are not meaningful to a child under five years old.

If possible, examine the forbidden object that interests the youngster together. Remembering the age of the child, try to find an explanation to show him what the danger is.

If you need to take something away from your toddler, offer something to replace it, but always with something new or interesting. In most cases, conflict can be avoided.

It is advisable for adults involved in the upbringing of a child to talk about the limits allowed, so as the toddler grows, he or she will not be confused: if dad considers this acceptable, why does grandma forbid it? Do not do this in the presence of the toddler.

Even when being guided by safety considerations, do not outlaw several things to the child, all in a row. This can destroy the child's desire for initiative or cause them excessive nervousness.

A child's desire to touch something with his hands or to taste it is not always due to mischief (as sometimes it seems to parents). This is the normal desire that a child has to know the world around him and to gain their own experiences..

If you treat them with respect, you can find many ways to manage his or her behavior. But, although you cannot do without verbal correction, you should not criticize their personality. Instead, focus on the act itself.

Try not to say to a child: "You are bad!" Instead, say, "You did a bad thing!" Even if your toddler does not understand everything, your attitude towards him and your tone of voice can make clear the meaning of what is happening.

Analyze the reasons for the conflicts that arise: is it possible that you are annoyed by seeing in your child a character trait that you have been trying to rid of yourself of for a long time?

When children are happy with everything, they usually behave well, but sometimes they unconsciously want to push the limits. At this time, it seems to parents that the child is testing their patience.

Often, bad behavior is a way to attract attention. The child may try to establish himself as being in opposition to the adults with whom they constantly communicates. If you see the child is very enthusiastic in an activity, try not to interrupt them, even if it is time to eat or sleep.

Help them finish their "business," and then suggest whatever next steps are on the agenda. The child will get used to finishing what he is doing.

The most sensible way to resist hysterics and fits, if they become habitual, is to ignore them. Stay calm and kind with your child, but firmly insist on your authority, and in the end, your toddler will understand that lying on the floor in hysterics is not the best way to win an argument.

It is not necessary to send a child to another room, especially if you are not sure about their safety. Go about your affairs, talk about other problems with your loved ones, and let the toddler remain in your field of vision. If, after some time, the child is ready for dialogue, do not reproach him for what took place a few minutes ago.

Sometimes a child needs some help to stop the hysteria.

Each family has its own ways of settling disobedience, based on their experience of communicating with the child.

Chapter 2:   How to Stimulate Good Behavior in Children

Educating our children was not easy. So, I went after tips on how to encourage good behavior in children, without having to punish and scold every second.

Stimulating good behavior in children is one of the best ways to impose limits, without having to apply punishments constantly. The only problem is how to do that. In most cases, our little ones tested our limits and seemed to do anything but obey.

Here are ways to stimulate good behavior:

Be the Example

Being an example is the most effective way we must teach our children anything—both good and bad. Here are a few examples of what you can do for your child to learn.

Catch your child's attention when you split snacks with your husband, or when you must wait in the bank queue, pointing out that adults also have to share and wait too.

Realize the Good Behavior

If you are like any parent in the world, when your child is behaving well, you leave them playing alone and take advantage of the time to do what you must attend to. But when your child is behaving badly, you direct all your attention to him to resolve the situation. Your attention is what kids most want, so to get this attention, sometimes children will behave badly. This is completely counterintuitive for us, but it is useful to understand this dynamic.

Understand the Stage of Development

This tip is easy to understand. Each child has a behavior; however, you cannot expect a child of three to act as the same as a child who is ten. That is, do not try to go to a three-hour lunch with your little boy, hoping he will be quiet for the whole lunch. We do not want a two-year-old child to put everything in his mouth. Each age has a phase, and it is of no use wanting to demand different behavior from a child.

Have Appropriate Expectations

Parents have high expectations. This is not wrong when expectations are possible. For example, do not expect a tired child to behave well, or a one-month-old baby to sleep through the night.

Create Structure and Routine

A child with a structured routine tends to behave better. They know what to expect and are used to it. A child with a routine feels safe and thus lives more calmly. A child without a routine has a sense of insecurity that will be disruptive. Use your time wisely: provide structure in order to educate and encourage good behavior.

Understand That the Bad Behavior Worked So Far

If throwing tantrums and disobeying worked for them to obtain your attention thus far, changing this behavior will take time. They will have to realize and understand that you will no longer pay attention to them when they behave badly, but will when they behave appropriately.

Instilling good behavior practices in young children is a must for any responsible parent, but sometimes it can also be quite complicated and laborious. However, beginning to instill this type of behavior, as early as possible, will help build a good foundation for the child's behavior and attitudes in the future. It is necessary to be aware that in the first years of life, children are like sponges, and results will be better if you begin to show them early and direct them to appropriate behaviors of life in society.

Here are some more ideas to help parents with the task of encouraging good behavior in their children.

Models to Follow

Children tend to mirror the behaviors of parents and those with whom they coexist more closely. Therefore, be careful about your behaviors and language used when the child is around, to avoid misunderstanding ideas and misconceptions about how you should behave towards others. This includes talking and behaving politely to both your partner and family, as well as to the child. Try to avoid loud, unstructured arguments when the child is around. We do not mean you cannot disagree with your spouse, because the child must also be aware that this can exist. But try to have the arguments always controlled and civil around children.

Be Firm

Parents should be affectionate, but still adamant about instilling discipline in their children. It is important that children know how to respect their parents, even when they do not get what they want. Understanding when to say no, at the right time, is an important step in their education.

Establishing Limits

It is fundamental to establish limits, rules, and consequences for unwanted behavior. Increase limits on children to be able to distinguish right from wrong. They need to know what is not acceptable, and a clear understanding of what makes it wrong, so that there is no doubt in the child's mind about the behaviors to adopt.

You started tracking your child's progress long before he left the warmth of your belly: In the tenth week, the heart began beating; on the twenty-fourth week, the hearing developed and they listened to your voice; in the thirtieth week, they began to prepare for childbirth. Now that he or she is in your arms, you are still eager to keep up with all the signs of your little one's development and worry that he might be left behind. Nonsense! Excessive worry will not help at all, so take your foot off the accelerator and enjoy each phase. Your child will realize all the fundamental achievements of maturity. They will learn to walk, talk, potty train—and when you least expect it—they will be riding a bicycle alone (with no training wheels!). They will do it all; but only in their time.

Stop taking developmental milestones so seriously. For example, your seven-month-old son will be able to sit alone, and at age three, will be able to ride a tricycle. Consider what is expected for each age for reference only. The best thing to do is to set aside the checklist of the abilities your child needs to develop and play together a lot. There is no better way to connect with and develop your child than through playtime.

Bonding & Trust

Establishing relationships of trust is important for the development of the child. The first people they build trust with is the parents. For this, one factor is essential: never lie. If the child goes to the doctor to take a vaccine, do not even think about saying that you are just going for a walk. If he asks if the injection will hurt, be honest and say, yes it will, but only for a short moment. The experts are all in agreement: explain everything. Tell them they are going to get wet; it is going to hurt; they will be cold, etc., so they know what to expect and learn to trust in what you say.

Congratulate your child when he is good at something, encouraging him to continue. If scolding is necessary, pay close attention to how to do it. Saying: "What you did was naughty," is quite different from saying: "You are naughty!" Do not let the child think that the criticized trait is part of their personality, so they will not incorporate this trait into their self-image.

Chapter 3: Positive Parenting Strategies For Toddlers

When you use positive reinforcement, you are trying to further encourage good behaviors, by making sure that your child sees that they are worthwhile. Children, like most people, are typically driven by positivity. We enjoy positive interactions with ourselves and with other people, and because of that, it is important to maintain that sort of positivity, as much as you can. You may have to, for example, make sure that you offer good, gentle encouragement to your child when they do something.

Positive reinforcement works by you offering a reward of some sort when your child behaves in a way that is constructive or beneficial to you and those around you. You will do this by making sure that you are always focusing on how much you can praise anything that is positive. While many people may believe that you need harsh punishment to create a well-disciplined child, you do not actually have to. You can create that good discipline in other ways such as ensuring that, at the end of the day, your child is taught that positivity is always the best policy.

Positive reinforcement can occur in many ways. You could, for example, offer your child heavy praise the first time he or she does something important or that was supposed to happen. You could use positive reinforcement to give your child a reward when they do something good as well. You may, for example, offer up stickers in return for meeting expectations, rather than creating a punishment in response to not meeting them.

When you do this, you motivate your child to do what he or she needs to do. Think about it—when you are told to do something, you probably do not really want to do it. Your toddler is no different. He does not want to pick up his toys because it is boring. There are other things that your child wants to do, such as playing, coloring, or watching television. Anything would be better.

When this happens, the best way to approach the situation is to figure out some way that you can ensure that you encourage your child to meet expectations. You could, for example, decide that you will implement that sticker chart. You are going to be praising your child and giving them something that they like. If they do not meet expectations, they do not get punished. They do not get told to go sit in time out. Rather, they do not get their sticker for the day, and that can be enough to motivate children to behave better in the future next time. Your child will not like having that sticker lost and will be more likely to move forward in the first place.

This works because you are primarily encouraging your child to want to do something, as opposed to teaching avoidance of something else. You are teaching your child that they need to do what you are asking because they need to avoid that negativity, not because they need to do it because it needs to be done. Because of that, particularly for things that are not going to be the end of the world, such as not picking up blocks or other toys, you should try to step away from the punishment side. Instead, think of things as natural consequences and positive reinforcement.

If your child does something wrong that is going to hurt someone, then you need to intervene. If you see that your child is, for example, spinning with a plastic bag over his head or playing with the curtain cords, you know that you need to intervene. You know that you need to avoid natural consequences, due to the fact that those natural consequences, in that instance, are going to be potentially irreversible.

When you use positive reinforcement to help mitigate tantrums, you make your child feel like cleaning and following the rules are pleasant. You make your child want to do what he or she is doing, and because your child wants to follow along, there should be fewer instances of tantrums. When you want to see the best possible results, you are going to want to make obedience pleasant and enjoyable.

Some ways that you can add in positive reinforcement with your child include the following:

- Implement a sticker chart for daily responsibilities
- Offer praise at certain increments when they are doing something—for example, offer a high five after every ten blocks that they pick up
- Offer a compliment when you catch your child doing something well
- Give a hug for completing a task
- Pay attention when your child is doing what they should.

Chapter 4: Communicating with Your Child

Communication is key in any relationship, and the one you have with your child is no different. The period from ages one through four years of age are vital to your toddler's emerging language and social skills. Parent-child communication during this stage of development is all about effective interaction, modelling communicative behaviors, and fostering confidence, safety, and self-development.

One thing to remember about communicating with your toddler is that it is a dynamic, two-way interaction. One reaches out, the other responds. As you and your toddler learn to interact in increasingly responsive and effective ways, he will develop an increased sense of safety, confidence, empathy, and self-determination.

Let us consider some of the key components of effective communication.

Effective Communication: Talking

The way that a parent speaks communicates much more than simply words. When you engage verbally with your toddler, you are modelling how a conversation works, including important skills, such as listening, empathy, and taking turns.

Talking to your toddler in ways that are too aggressive or too passive can have negative consequences on their emotional and social development, as well as detract from the potential benefits of teaching moments and healthy discipline. Rather, parents should speak firmly but kindly, as they seek to communicate with their toddlers.

Let us consider some important tips for talking in ways that your toddler can understand:

Tip 1: Use eye contact. When talking with your toddler, do not expect them to listen or understand if you are just talking at them. Set aside any distractions, make eye contact, and let yourself connect fully with your little one

Eye contact will help your toddler to pay attention to what you are saying and stay engaged in the conversation. It will also help bolster their sense of personhood by making it clear that you are interested in them.

Tip 2: Speak to them by name. Using your toddler's name while talking with them is another way to keep them focused on the conversation. This will give them a sense of importance, as a part of the conversation. It is especially important to use names when validating or when you are trying to let them know that you approve or disapprove. For example: "Wow Johnny, that sounds so frustrating," or "I love how you shared with your sister, Alex," or "We do not throw food David—please stop."

Tip 3: Do not yell. Once you start yelling, chances are that your toddler's behavior will become worse, either right then and there, or manifest in the next day or week. Yelling sets a poor example for your toddler and is likely to cause them stress that could become damaging. You may also frighten them, further adding to their anxiety and fueling further misbehavior, as they try to cope.

Instead, speak in a calm but firm voice. If needed, take a moment to breathe and calm down before speaking.

Tip 4: Be assertive, but not aggressive. Sometimes kids misinterpret our responses and may not realize that we are serious about a limit or may think that we are engaging in play. Be clear about the purpose of your communications by using an assertive tone and body language when appropriate. However, do not mistake assertiveness for aggression. Assertiveness effectively communicates ideas and expectations; aggressiveness communicates danger, fear, and dislike.

Tip 5: Smile. Babies and toddlers are particularly responsive to facial expressions. As you no doubt discovered during the first year, sometimes a well-directed smile is all that it takes to brighten up a discontented baby. The same holds true for toddlers. Offering smiles during a conversation lets your toddler know that you enjoy talking with them and that the conversation is meant to be fun.

Tip 6: Minimize the use of "no." While some limits will certainly focus on what your toddler should do, many will be focused on what they should not do. Hearing no repeatedly throughout the day can be exhausting for your little one. Try to talk to him in positive terms that model reasoning. For example, instead of saying, "No Michael! Do not throw your food," you might try, "Hmmm, throwing our food makes the floor sticky. Let us try saving it for later instead."

Tip 7: Do not talk too much. When speaking, keep it simple. Toddlers have short attention spans and talking too much will likely cause your toddler to lose interest. For example, one day, two-year-old Jimmy threw his toy car straight at the window in his bedroom. His mom responded by saying, 'Now Jimmy, you cannot throw your toy car at the window because if you end up breaking the window we're going to have to buy a new one, and that costs a lot of money. Besides, throwing things is dangerous—what if you hurt someone? How do you think it would feel? Do you think it is nice..." At this point, Jimmy has stopped listening. His mother is using too many words, discussing people that are not even present, and speaking in terms that a two-year-old cannot follow or relate to. Instead, she might say something like: "Jimmy, do not throw your toys in the house. Throwing is for outside." At two years of age, short, direct explanations of not more than two or three sentences are the most likely to result in understanding.

Tip 8: Use good manners. Using "please" and "thank you" will model good manners for your toddler, as well as help her to see that kids and adults alike deserve respect in conversation.

Tip 9: Ask questions. Asking open-ended questions is a great way to show interest in your toddler and encourage their participation in the conversation. When trying to encourage interaction, avoid questions that can be answered with a short yes/no. Instead of asking, "Did you go to the park with Grandma?" ask, "What did you do at the park?"

Tip 10: Do not limit the conversation to directions. Finally, do not just use talk to give your little one directions or feedback. Their language skills are growing a mile a minute at this age, and they are learning that language can be used for all kinds of purposes. Support this growth and create positive interaction patterns by asking them about their day, their opinions, asking them to tell stories, solve problems out loud, etc. Responses will be limited at first but need not be any less enjoyable. You will be astounded by how quickly your toddler's language develops in just a few short years.

Effective Communication: Listening

Listening goes hand in hand with talking. Being a good listener will encourage your toddler to talk and help them develop good communication skills. Remember, effective communication with your toddler is dynamic and interactive, which means modelling both talking and listening abilities.

Listening serves several communicative purposes, including gathering information, opening the door for empathy, building relationships, giving respect, and gaining perspective. Listening will help you to understand what is going on in your little one's mind and heart, letting you relate to them better, as you help them solve problems.

Tip 1: Ask for details. When your toddler tells you about what happened at church or that her baby doll feels sad, show that you are listening by asking for more details. What happened first? Second? Third? Why is the baby doll sad? How will you make her happy? In addition to showing that you are listening and interested, such questions elicit a new language and help your toddler to practice important cognitive functions such as recall, mental modelling, and problem solving.

Tip 2: Pay attention. In today's world, multitasking has become a way of life, even when it is unnecessary. To show your toddler that you are listening and engaged, set aside devices such as phones or tablets and give them your full attention.

Tip 3: Use active listening. Active listening refers to listening that is purposeful and fully engaged. During active listening, you are fully focused on what is being said. Body language cues, including eye contact, mirroring facial expressions, and an attentive posture all contribute to active listening. When you listen actively, your toddler will be more likely to feel that what they have to say is important, and they will be encouraged to speak more.

Tip 4: Be physically interactive. High fives, hugs, and gestures are all great ways to show that you are listening and interested in what your toddler is saying. Getting bodies involved will also make the conversation more engaging and meaningful.

Tip 5: Give unconditional love. Toddlers seriously lack impulse control and often do not know how to express themselves in socially appropriate ways. They may speak out of anger and even say things like, "I hate you," or "You are ugly." Remember, do not take it personally! No matter how your toddler speaks to you, or what the content of their message is, make sure that they always know that you love them, no matter what. Unconditional love creates a safe space, in which toddlers are able to speak freely and make mistakes, without fear of losing your love or affection. This freedom will do wonders for their language skills, confidence, and trust in you as a parent..

Chapter 5: Disciplining Your Toddler

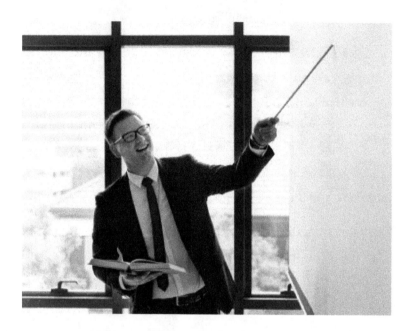

No doubt, you would like to have a well-behaved child. You may even be feeling pressure from family members, friends, and strangers you meet on the street to make sure your mini-me stays polite and quiet. Here is the good news: you can have a well-behaved child. The bad news: you cannot have one all of the time. By the very nature of human brain development, our children require time, patience, and guidance to learn how to treat others with respect and regulate their own emotional states.

What Is Discipline?

How do you make a child behave? The answer may be shocking: you do not. He alone is able to choose to modify his behavior within the scope of his current developmental capabilities. But you have a lot of power as his parent. You can help him make the choice to comply or cooperate with your requests, and you can teach him about the behavioral expectations for different situations in your culture. He needs discipline. To use the transitive verb to bring home the point, he needs to be disciplined by you.

Parenting experts still debate about what effective discipline for young children looks like, and there are many techniques you can try. Punishment may immediately come to mind, but routine spanking smacking, isolating, or taking away possessions, privileges, or experiences from a child can have unintended consequences later in life.

A better approach to disciplining your child is to use techniques that enrich his ability to make judgments. This does not mean letting him do whatever he wants. While he is a toddler, you are the one responsible for making any major decisions that you feel are in his best interest. Since a toddler lacks the cognitive ability to use reason or logic to solve problems or decide what behavior is appropriate in any given situation, you will be coaching him, step-by-step. His budding independence will emerge by making simple, meaningful choices at first. When he releases his big emotions and loses control, you will offer your support by empathizing and giving him the boundaries he needs to feel safe and loved.

Setting Realistic Goals

Parents often have expectations for behavior that are not realistic given the ages of their children. This contains developmental information, with suggestions for realistic behavioral expectations, for each age and stage. This will help you know whether the technique you are choosing will support your short or long-term goals for your child's growth and development.

Short-Term Goals

There will be times when you need to set a limit, and either commit to enforcing it quickly, or let go of your ideal routine. Here are a few examples of some common short-term goals related to behavioral issues.

- Compliance for the sake of safety

- Getting a good night's sleep

- Using good manners

- Stopping the whining

Long-Term Goals

You might start by thinking about what you consider to be your own strengths and the experiences that helped you develop them. Also think about your family and community values. Which would you consider a high priority?

Disciplining your often unreasonable, highly emotional toddler can be frustrating. To remind yourself of these long-term goals, you might even keep this list in a place where you will see it every day.

Temperament And Behavior

Your parenting style will have a significant influence on how your child behaves and perceives her place in the world, but it is not the only factor by far. Many people assume that a child's personality is always the direct result of how permissive or dictatorial the parent is. This is a myth. Your child is a unique and valuable person, born with a predisposition toward certain traits that developed in utero and continued to be formed by their experiences throughout early childhood.

In a revolutionary 1970 study of infant reactions to stimuli, Alexander Thomas, Stella Chess, and Herbert G. Birch determined that a child's personality is formed by the constant interplay of temperament and environment. The nine temperament traits identified in this study give us insight into why children raised in similar environments may behave differently from one another.

Activity level: This trait refers to your child's general energy level. A high-energy child can be a handful with all the squirming and wiggling, while a more sedentary child can be hard to motivate physically, as quiet, calm activities are preferred. If your toddler is constantly climbing the furniture, running in circles, and popping in and out of bed at night, provide ample access to the outdoors on a daily basis so that their muscles have the freedom to move. Indoors, focus on ways to safely meet their need to stretch and explore independently.

Rhythmicity: How predictable is your child's natural, biological rhythm? Some children will eat, sleep, and have bowel movements with extreme regularity. For them, a predictable schedule is a comfortable one and largely self-determined. Other children show much more irregularity, which can complicate meals, naps, and toilet learning. Parental intervention and flexibility are necessary to avoid conflict.

Distractibility: Is your child easily distracted by outside influences? A child with high distractibility will often be satisfied when you exchange an unsafe object for a safe toy or when you sing a song while performing an unappealing task, such as buckling a car seat or changing a diaper. A child who is less willing to be distracted will not stop fussing until the task has been completed.

Initial response: When confronted with a new situation, such as a new person, food, toy, or activity, how eagerly does your child embrace the new experience? Some children approach them with ease, immediately interacting and engaging impulsively. Others are slow to warm up, taking time to get comfortable and assess the situation. When you introduce your child to a new person, such as a babysitter, they may prefer to sit quietly in your lap observing for a while before interacting. However, the withdrawal of some children from new experiences is much more dramatic and requires considerable adult encouragement and patience. A child with an initial negative response to new situations will cry, hide, or run away. They will need emotional support and lots of time to adjust to new experiences.

Adaptability: This refers to your child's ability to adjust over time to new experiences, routines, or expectations. If your child is adaptable in temperament, transitioning from one activity to another will not be a big deal. Settling into a new schedule may take some time, but you will not typically encounter much resistance from your child. Other children will react adversely to new routines, as evidenced by tantrums, defiance, or anxious behaviors. These children will benefit from more gradual shifts in routine, rather than dramatic ones.

Attention span and persistence: Does your child concentrate on a single activity for a long time? Do they continue to repeat and practice new skills, despite any obstacles in her way? The child with higher levels of attention and persistence will not give up easily when asked to perform tasks that are initially frustrating. On the other hand, if you interrupt this same child to ask them to move on to another activity, you may be met with resistance and an inflexible attitude. If your child has a shorter attention span and less persistence, they may need a more step-by-step approach, reminders, and visual cues to help her complete difficult tasks.

The intensity of reaction: How strongly does your child show their emotions? Very intense children may be labeled as overdramatic, celebrating with extreme exuberance when excited and sobbing or tantrum over minor disappointments. Children with lower levels of intensity may smile or cry, but in general, their reaction to events will be much more subdued by comparison.

Sensory threshold: In response to varied physical sensations, does your child react positively, negatively, or not at all? Some children are sensitive and easily overwhelmed by sensory input, such as noise, light, or textures, which makes crowded, noisy places difficult to navigate. Others will react in the opposite way and will seek out more stimulation on purpose.

Quality of mood: Does your child tend to be cheerful and upbeat or have a distrustful and serious demeanor? Your child's moods will, of course, vary from day to day, but in general, most children lean toward a more positive or a more negative emotional state.

Age-Appropriate Discipline

Your child's general temperament may stay fairly constant from infancy, but the natural course of human development is not a steady path. As your child grows older, his needs, interests, and behaviors will shift, sometimes dramatically, therefore, your discipline strategies must also cater to his present self, not to the child he was before.

Using the "distract and redirect" technique is often very effective and easy to implement for a one-year-old, even if your child's temperament is fairly low in distractibility. However, a few years later, this same technique is not likely to go over well, as four-year-olds have longer attention spans and a clearer understanding of how to follow the rules. At age three and above, most children are able to make the connection between their actions and the natural consequences, but not before. Sparking the imagination is a technique that speaks especially to a four-year-old's proclivity for pretend play, while a one-year-old would just be confused.

Chapter 6:   Nine Methods for Toddler Discipline

Instilling discipline is a dilemma for most parents, especially the new ones. They look for the most effective approach to raise well-mannered and positive children, who are capable of coping up with the challenges in the real world.

Technically, there is no right or wrong approach, except the punitive ways that scar children for life.

Here are some simple methods that are widely used by parents all over the world:

1.   Commendation & Encouragement

Praise and encouraging words always bring positive outcomes, motivating toddlers to show good behavior. Giving your child small rewards or applause when he does something commendable will encourage him to continue improving his skills. Praising good behaviors will make him repeat the same thing, again and again, to gain your approval and praise.

2.   Rethinking

Changing the tone of your discourse or reframing your thoughts often results in a positive reaction. Instead of giving an instruction that uses "Do not do that," or "Get that," rethink your strategy to mirror a solicitation. It is better to use the phrases "Would you . . . If it is okay with you?"

Remember that your toddler is not a tiny you. It also helps to view things from their perspective. For instance, if they do not want to sit in the child car seat, you might say: "I know that you do really like sitting in your car seat, but it is almost like this seat belt that I have. They keep us both safe." In this manner, you are teaching him the importance of being safe by using proper tools.

3.   Disregard

Disregarding fits or tantrums intentionally sends a clear signal to your child that you are not affected by his behavior, and you will not succumb to his whims. To make it more effective, all other adults in your home must know this strategy to discipline and break the child's tantrum habits. It may seem harsh, but refraining to engage or respond to your child's temper tantrum is one of the keys to curb the habit.

Ignoring or looking the other way is an effective way to curb the child's habit of doing something naughty just to get your attention. Avoid meeting their eyes, glaring, or getting angry because it signifies your attention to them. You need to act like you are not disturbed by their behavior, making them realize that screaming or throwing tantrums will not make you yield to their desires.

4.   Break

It is also called a time-out, a popular technique most parents use to discipline their children. The idea is to send them to a certain "cozy spot" in your home, a particular place that is safe and free from stimulation or distraction, and let them reflect on their behavior. It is important that you can see them and ensure their safety. After a certain amount of time, talk about what happened, giving them time to explain and admit their misdeed.

A good rule is setting a time limit must correspond to the age of the child, so if your child is two years old, enforce a two-minute break. However, use this method sparingly and avoid making them feel isolated or alone.

5.   Substitute & Distraction

If your child has a habit of hitting something inside the house, like banging their toy on the table, distract them before they can do it. You can attract their attention by showing them something. Young children are easy to distract because they usually have a short attention span. You can also substitute their toys, redirecting them into something more interesting.

Toddlers do not understand why they are being disciplined. Divert their attention with another activity or toy that will interest them. Calling their name aloud grabs his attention, then once their eyes are fixed on you, show them something that will compel them to come to you.

6.   Offer Decisions

Letting your child take part in simple decision-making, like what color of the shirt they want to wear, gives them a sense of pride and control. It boosts their confidence and lessens the occurrences of power struggles. By involving them in the process, you ease the transition and make them proud of making a choice.

These last three methods should be avoided as much as possible.

7.   Surrendering to fits of rage

Your little child will be persistent and throw fits of rage, to make you give in to their demands. If you yield the first time, it becomes a ticket for them to attempt another try. It is the toddler's control strategy, and they can be prevented by not yielding to their unreasonable requests that will compromise their health and safety.

8.   Raising your voice. When is it appropriate?

Some parents admit that, at one time or another, they yell at their children. Studies show that yelling is one of the discipline techniques that can make behavior issues worse, undermining the parent and child bond. It also loses its effectiveness over time, when your child begins to tune you out as you do it regularly.

When is yelling necessary? Expressing your emotions aloud can be positive for you and your child, helping them develop empathy and realize that they have upset you. However, be mindful of your language. Instead of "you" statements, use "I" statements like: "I am feeling disappointed because you will not share your toys with your brother," rather than "You are not being nice!"

It is also necessary to be aware of your inner feelings and behavior. Sometimes, you bellow out because you are in a bad mood or tired, and not because your child has done something awfully wrong.

9.   Punishment

Punishment in all forms, including spanking, caning, and beating is a big NO. It has been a tactic in the past, used by parents to control their children, but many studies showed that it caused long-term disdain and misery. Spanking, for example, even occasional, can lead to the development of childhood anxiety and causes your child to think that it is okay to hit others .

Children learn to be afraid of the consequences when caught, but do it anyway when you are not present. If you say, "Do not let me catch you doing it again, or you will be grounded!" they may interpret the act as not inappropriate, but they just need to be careful, so that you will not catch them doing it. The result does not resolve the behavior problem and becomes ineffective in helping the child make better choices or learn self-control. There is also a consistent result in various surveys that punishment pushes children to spend more time in avoidance behavior and being rebellious.

Chapter 7:   Dealing with Difficult Toddlers

We have established that toddlers can be difficult, thus the need to train them comes in. We should not just claim that they will understand once they are older: it may be too hard for you to stop the behaviors once they are more mature. They are toddlers: they are not unintelligent, and they know the difference between right and wrong. This may not align well with your thinking, but an open mind will help you think from a different perspective.

Four Common Struggles Toddlers May Have

Toddlers do not understand the logic of waiting and the logic behind having everything they want. They no nothing or little about self-control, and in a nutshell, he/she may be having a hard time balancing his/her needs with what you are providing as a parent or caregiver. Toddlers can be difficult; they can be unpredictable too. Here are four common situations your child could be struggling with:

1. They say no when they mean yes. This happens when you are offering them a favorite treat.

2. They have a meltdown anytime you fail to understand their words.

3. They do not want any substitute. The blue pajamas or nothing else: even though they may not be washed, or even after offering them the purple ones.

4. They act out when frustrated, giving up everything when angry.

What is listed above are only charades that toddlers assume to manage strong feelings. Since they are new to almost everything, they lack command over what controls them and how they can leverage it. They soon find out that they have vocal powers, and that is when the crying, shouting, and yelling increases. They may want to enact different rackets, to see how they sound, and the reactions of adults around them to such noise. They impulsively go into an activity without much forethought. It is essential for you to know that there exists a peculiarity in each child. They react differently to different situations; in fact, you can even place a label on them. Most times you can start with some funny names like bubbly, daredevil, determined, stubborn, cautious, adventurous etc. Some challenging toddler behavior is developmentally correct: they may be defiant, bossy, sassy, or impulsive, but they are just byproduct of what the child needs: independence.

Six Difficult Behaviors And Their Practical Solutions

Unfortunately, some bad behaviors are common among toddlers. Here are the six difficult behaviors and their practical solutions:

Aggression, Hitting and Biting

Aggressive behavior is normal for toddlers: do not be surprised. Provided below are practical solutions on what you are to do when you come across an aggressive toddler.

- Make sure you keep your cool: keeping your cool shows how controlled you are, do not yell at the child when he/she is in the aggressive mode. If you tell your child they are bad, you are just getting them riled up.

- Let your limits be clear: your reply to your aggressive toddler should be immediate.

- Alternatives should be taught: explain to him or her briefly on the consequences of his or her last action. It is natural to have angry feelings, but it is not okay to show them by kicking, hitting, or biting. They should apologize after lashing out someone, for any reason. Such an apology should be sincere, even though it may look insincere to you. With this, the lesson will sink in.

- Keep your toddler active: if you notice your child is a high spirited one, give them plenty of unstructured time, outdoors preferably. This gives them much-needed time to burn off that abundance of energy.

- Get help if you need it: speak to a pediatrician if you notice that your child's aggression is atrocious. But, this should be when you have noticed some or all of the following features:

  o   Your child finds it easy to attack adults.

  o   He or she enjoys making other children upset or frightened.

  o   He or she remains aggressive for a week after you have tried all you could.

Interrupting

Nothing can be so exasperating than a child who intrudes every time you are chatting with a friend. Toddlers do not really interrupt with words all the time but also with their actions. That is because they always seek attention from their parents and may be jealous if a friend or an adult is getting all of your focus. In this aspect, it is your fault. You can do the following:

- Chose the right locale for your meetings. A place where your child can freely play while you talk with the adult. A park with a sandbox is one option.

- Teach your children polite behavior. A good way to teach them is by reading them some books like *The Berenstain Bears Forget Their Manners*, by Stan and Jan Berenstain or *The Bad Good Manners Book*, by Babette Cole; *Manners By Aliki* and *What Do you Say, Dear?* by Sesyle Joslin. Any book on good manners you can lay your hands on. Read it to them every day.

- Schedule your phone calls. You would not want your child to disturb you while you are on a call, so make necessary preparations.

Lying

First, why do children lie? They have an active imagination, and they are very forgetful. These cute angels may also have what we call angel syndrome. A child who thinks that his parents believe he can do no wrong, and would not do wrong on purpose. When asked, a lie comes to mind. Toddlers do lie, and it is natural for them to do so. How can you stop this?

- Always encourage truth-telling. You should not be mad at your child when he or she tells you the truth: instead you should be happy. Show your child that honesty pays off.

- You should not accuse your child for any reason. Your comments and remarks should help your child, not put him down.

- Do not weigh your child down with too many expectations. He or she would not understand. They are children, toddlers not adults.

- Build your trust. Trust your child and make sure they know it, and do not puncture that trust.

Pulling Hair

To begin with, pulling hair, biting, pinching, hitting etc. are ways your child showcases his feelings or applies control over what seems to be his immediate environment (his body). Roberts, a professor of clinical psychology at Idaho State University in Pocatello claims that: "A child might be pulling the hair to make bad things go away." For whatever reason, you should take the following steps when this happens:

- Stop the behavior as soon as it starts. When you catch them holding a fistful of hair, stop them immediately. Hold their hand firmly while you keep repeating this sentence, "We do not pull hair. Pulling hair hurts."

- Take time to give a detailed explanation, but make sure it is very brief. You should start by asking him or her: "What did you do that was wrong?" After the reply, make use of that opportunity to tell them that pulling hair only hurts themselves and others.

- You should not be guilty of the same offense. Do not pull your child's hair if you do not want them to pull it also.

Running Away

A toddler running away can be quite humorous. Like really? Where do they think they are going? But you have to be careful when this happens outdoors, especially on the sidewalk. Why do they run? Toddlers like the feeling of being free and running around; you can encourage it, as long as you can control where they run. You cannot stop this; you can only control it:

- Stay close to them: it should be okay if you to look ahead for dangers when they are running.
- Show them where they can run and where they cannot. Allow them to explore the safe areas
- Entertain your child.

Teasing

You may agree or not, teasing is just a part of life. It happens, and even toddlers are not excluded from it. It is really painful when toddlers are teased, and you should understand that as a parent. What can you do when a toddler is teased? This may not work well for toddlers, as they would require a verbal response. However:

- Your child should not respond. This could be hard, but it is a trick that can repel those guilty of the teasing offense.
- You can coach your child to "agree" with what the teaser is saying. He/she would look dumb when a child says, "I agree: I suck my thumb"
- Ask for help. Your child can ask for help from anyone or any adult around.

Chapter 8: Toddlers and Tantrums

To toddlers, everything is new. Your child does not realize that you need to work to earn money to trade for that cool new toy on the shelf—they just know that the toy is there, and they want it. They may realize that you hand over money or swipe a card when you pay, but that has no intrinsic value to the child—they do not understand that the money must be earned, so they do not understand why you cannot just hand over the toy.

Your toddler does not know how to communicate their reasoning for wanting the toy, nor does your toddler understand why you may be saying no to it—they just know that you have said no. They cannot properly have that sort of communication exchange with you when they are unable to properly work out their feelings on the matter. When they have no other way to communicate, they melt down. Their feelings are overwhelming. They simply melt down and cry because that is all that they know to do. They do not have the words that they need to look at you and say, "Yes, mother and father, I am quite frustrated with the fact that you took that great looking toy from me and told me that I could not have it. I really wish you would just let me have it, or at least give me a reason that makes sense to me. It is right there! I can touch it! It is not anyone else's toy, so why can I not have it?"

What Is A Tantrum?

Temper tantrums are frustrating. There is no way around it. However, they are not a majorly negative event—rather, they are learning experiences for everyone involved. Your child does not know better than to throw those tantrums. They happen when your child is feeling incredibly emotional, but is unsure about how to handle those big emotions that are roiling around inside him or her. For that reason, you should approach tantrums with grace and understanding—you should be willing and able to recognize that your child is not throwing this massive fit to hurt you, but rather because he or she feels entirely out of control.

Tantrums can range greatly from kicking and screaming to hitting or holding one's breath. Some children, particularly the stubborn ones, will hold their breath until they finally end up passing out due to oxygen deprivation. While alarming to watch happen at the moment, it is not putting your child at any real risk, and your child's body will take control before he or she can do any real, lasting harm.

Most often, these tantrums happen between the ages of one and three. Everything is new to your child—he or she may be learning how to interact with the world. There is the development of the concept of autonomy during this age as well—your child is finally beginning to recognize that he or she is their own independent person. Your child wants to interact and do so much, but they cannot communicate. They may want to impulsively do things that you know are harmful, such as jumping off a counter, and when you stop them, they throw a fit. They cannot comprehend the reasoning behind why you say no at this point in time, and they find that they get overwhelmed by that frustration, disappointment, anger, or sadness that follows.

Redirection To Tame Tantrums

Perhaps one of the best skills that you have on you as a parent is the ability to redirect during a tantrum. They are throwing a fit, usually due to their emotional side of their brains being on autopilot, at that point in time. When the emotional side is running rampant and taking control of the situation, we are not making good decisions. We are acting in ways that are impulsive, and with that impulsiveness often comes all sorts of other problems as well. Our decisions can wind up having all sorts of unintended repercussions that we were not ready to deal with.

You can show them something entirely different from what they are currently focused on to sort of stopping them in their tracks. You see this often with young babies: you may shake a rattle in front of him or her in hopes of distracting from crying, or you may offer a pacifier or a bottle. However, by the toddler years, some people stop this process of attempting to redirect. The stop is attempting to redirect their children just due to the fact that, at the end of the day, they expect that their older children are more capable of coping with the changes that come with growing up. However, the tactics that you use with an infant really are not much different than you would use with a toddler that is still learning to navigate the world around them. It will come with time, effort, and skill.

Redirection can happen in many different ways as well. Primarily, however, it is the same—you are going to be redirecting from a negative situation into a positive one, in some way, shape, or form. For example, let us say that your toddler just knocked down his blocks for the umpteenth time and is now throwing a fit. He kicked at the blocks and threw one across the room. You can redirect here by trying to show something else or do something else instead. You may say, for example: "Throwing blocks hurts people. We do not throw blocks. Would you like to play cars or throw a ball outside instead?" You are not reprimanding your child. You are not shaming or punishing your child. You are simply calmly trying to redirect his or her attention instead.

Give Controlled Choices

When you have a toddler that is throwing fits because he or she wants to exert some semblance of control, you have quite an easy solution already lined up for you: Give your child the illusion of choice. Think about it—if you let your child think that he or she has a choice to make, you are going to eliminate the problem altogether because your child will be satisfied. You give your child the illusion that he or she has some semblance of control and suddenly, your child will be much more agreeable in general.

Think about it this way—what your toddler wants is to make a decision. Your toddler is beginning to recognize autonomy, and because of that, your toddler wants to exercise it. This is precisely why the word no becomes so prevalent with young children. It is oftentimes one of the first words that children learn, due to the fact that children typically want to use it.

You will know when this is the case—you will ask if your child wants to do something, only to be met with that dreaded, "No!!" It will happen, over and over again. Instead, your child will resist, scream, and fight back. When that happens, you can usually direct your child out of this mindset.

You have to give your child a choice. It doesn't have to be any choice—you should always make sure that whatever it is that you are asking your child to do, or something they want to do, is what you can live with at the end of the day. You have to make sure that whatever you are willing to offer is something that you are willing to accept. This works very simply—it gives the illusion of choice. However, when you do this, you still maintain all of the control.

Imagine, for example, that your toddler refuses to eat his or her vegetables. You experience this every night—you have the same battle—you make a vegetable, and your child throws a fit.

Remember, children are not capable of thinking in the same way that you are—they do not think ahead. They do not recognize everything that they need in the same way that parents do. They do not see why they cannot logically walk out of the house, on a summer evening, wearing five different layers of clothing. They need boundaries. They need limitations. They need guidance. All of that can be provided when you limit choices. You make sure that the choice is a good choice for your child, encouraging independence and empowering your child to learn what is the right option, without overwhelming him or her.

Chapter 9: Establishing Limits and Rules

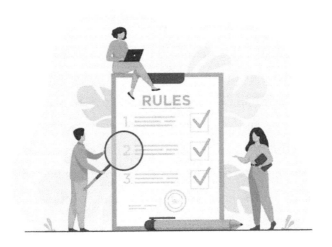

Boundaries are a framework: a guideline that shows which behavior is acceptable and which is not, and must be clear, concrete, and well defined. When setting boundaries, it is important to be consistent, because that way, the child will know that the boundaries cannot be negotiated at different times and places. The child must understand that the boundaries you set for them are not something that is disputable or variable. The boundaries must be set, and within that framework, certain rules have to be followed. However, that does not mean that those rules need to be overly strict.

It is clear that growing up within positively defined limits is the best way for a child to gradually develop life skills and learn to deal with everyday challenges. Therefore, those limits need to be set up in a timely manner. It is also important to make sure to establish an atmosphere of love and acceptance before, and not after, problems arise.

The Difference Between A Children's Wants and Needs

When a child asks for permission to do something, the parent needs to determine the answer, based on the values and rules that they and their family hold. Certainly, before we say no to something, we need to think carefully, so as not to constantly change the rules, but at the same time, it is necessary to keep in mind that the boundaries are not set in stone, but that with time, they need to be changed and adjusted, according to the developmental age of a child.

When setting boundaries, we must know how to distinguish children's wants and needs. Children are often unaware of their needs, but they always know what they want. If parents just satisfy children's wishes, then the children will be the ones deciding what is good for them, something for which they are, of course, not ready for. We must know when we need to say no, but not denying the child's basic needs for food, clothing, footwear, health, sleep, love, and social relations.

Rebellion Against the Rules

When we say no, children may become disappointed, sad, or angry, and begin to cry. This is a normal way for children to respond to frustration, and it is a necessary part of growing up. When children are angry and frustrated, we should never mock them; imitate them; blame them (from the second to the fifth year of a child's life, blame directly threatens his sense of personal worth and self-esteem), criticize; cajole; persuade them to feel guilty; or to stop expressing their emotions—and especially not to change their opinion. It is necessary to accept the child's feelings, to sympathize with them,   and to help them to direct their emotions and to remain consistent.

It is important not to give in when a child is pleading, crying, yelling, or in any way rebelling against the rules that you set. If we give in, the child will learn to use that kind of behavior when they want something and the next time: they will resort to it again. If they learn from their family that everything will go the way they want whenever they scream or cry, they will use the same kind of behavior in kindergarten, and that will make it much more difficult for the child to socialize.

When setting the boundaries, it is necessary to ensure that the child is heard and understood, so it is best to sit down with them, look them in the eye, and say what you want: in a simple and clear way that is understandable to them. You should never promise or threaten what you cannot fulfill. Do not give up because of the child's pressure ("Please, only this time!"), because normally, this will demonstrate to the child that you did not think out what you said. If you want to be flexible, do it before your child requests something.

Researchers once decided to collect evidence to show that parental affection benefits the welfare of children during their childhood, but in their research, they found that kisses and hugs from mom and dad mean even more than they thought. Scientists believe that greater self-confidence, better communication between parents and children, and less psychological and behavioral problems are linked to the warmth and attachment between parents and the child. This is one of the most important foundations of a parent-child relationship: tenderness, warmth, understanding, and trust.

Do you feel your stress and exhaustion disappear, when after a long day at work, you come home and hug and kiss your little ones? Children also feel that love and affection. Researchers have found that neglecting a child, which is linked to reduced attachment and love, can affect the child's physical and mental health for life, leading to negative consequences such as poor health. We know that children, regardless of their culture, need to feel loved. Children "absorb" the meaning of what their mothers and fathers are trying to do for them.

Can You Overdo Love? Yes, Sure You Can. But There Is A Solution: Be Moderate.

In child raising, setting personal limits is just as important as understanding, love, and support. When there are limits, children learn that they are responsible for what is happening to them, it helps them learn to self-regulate their feelings and behaviors, and helps them to be self-confident. These are essential skills that enable the child to achieve better success in school, and also to establish contact with peers and build friendships. Numerous studies show that an educational style in which support, acceptance, warmth and love are shown, and also in which there is a clear and consistent setting of boundaries and structure, and in which expectations are high, enables children to grow into self-confident, stable, and successful people, who cultivate quality relationships with others.

Why Is It Important for A Child to Learn How To Cope With Feelings Of Frustration, Sadness, And Anger?

These are skills that should be learned with the help of their parents. True, it is a difficult job and children need the outward support of adults. The smaller they are, the more leadership they need.

In order to have the boundaries that we set, make a positive impact on the emotional and social development of the child, the way in which these boundaries are set up is extremely important—they need to be set up clearly, consistently, and without punishment.

When setting boundaries, a key step is to respect the child's needs and feelings. When children have difficulty controlling emotions, describing the emotions to them is the first step to teach a child about what is happening to them. For example: "You were very angry because you couldn't watch the cartoon anymore, and you hit me. But I do not want to be hit because that hurts me."

In order for the limit to make sense to a child, you must explain to them a consequence. The most common consequences are natural consequences, that is, those related to what the child is doing. For example, if the child continues to play with the ball in the room after you have told him or her not to, the natural consequence is that you take the ball away. Do this without raising your voice. Simply put the ball away and tell your child that the apartment is not the place for such a type of game and that he can take the ball with him when you go to the park.

If a parent loses control when a child behaves badly and starts yelling, the little one usually responds with an outburst of anger, and the problem is doubled. Keep in mind that a child is just learning important life skills, and that you will best help him if you stay calm.

It is known that a lack of clear boundaries often leads to behavioral problems, so it is important to start creating healthy boundaries while children are still small. It is natural for children to try to push the limits and rules, as they develop their own understanding of themselves and learn how the world works.

Parents who provide limits for their children help them to develop moral principles. The goal of setting good limits is for the child to achieve self-control. Self-control, in turn, develops a solid character and an inner moral compass that further leads children to make good choices and be honest.

The boundaries should be set with as few negative emotions as possible. When a parent communicates calmly and clearly, there is less likelihood of the child being defiant. Children are perfect mirrors that reflect both positive and negative emotions. They usually do exactly what the parents themselves do, reflecting their aggravated state, not what they say. When parents consistently adhere to the boundaries and the consequences they have set, then children can more easily learn to respect others, build better self-control, develop the ability to tolerate frustration, and take responsibility for their actions.

Differences Between Boundaries, Orders, And Rules

Setting limits allows you to avoid conflicts between parent and child, while commands are based on penalties and negative consequences. Well-established boundaries are not based on the child's fear of the parent nor the fear of anger and punishment. They allow a child to experience positive and negative consequences in a safe environment of unconditional parental love. Also, such limits allow children to be responsible for their own behavior.

A child should not be blackmailed or threatened. It is better to praise them and allow some privileges for desirable and acceptable behavior. If a child behaves inappropriately and improperly, it is also very important to be sure that the child knows why this behavior was unacceptable before a certain privilege is taken away. Taking away a privilege must never mean taking away parental love or hindering the satisfaction of the child's developmental and emotional needs.

Children need guidance and direction in order to adopt family values, and the parents are the ones who make this possible. Parents provide a barrier between a child and the improper values which come at them from all sides, and parents take the responsibility for the child by setting clear, concrete, and well-defined boundaries which they stand behind firmly. After all, you cannot play a game if you do not know the rules. Boundaries are most effective when are put in place in an atmosphere of love, acceptance, and mutual respect.

Chapter 10: The Power of Empathy

Being an empathetic parent is the best gift a parent can give to their child. Your empathy for your child will let them understand that you actually "get them." Just like adults need someone to show confidence in them and acknowledge their feelings, so do young kids, especially toddlers. We need an understanding shoulder to lean on and cope with in our time of distress. That shoulder will only be supported when the person understands where we are coming from and what is the reason for our present situation.

Toddlers are no different. They need us, their parents, to be those understanding shoulders for them. We can become such strong support for them only by showing empathy. It is essential for kids that we understand them and their needs. For toddlers, their emotional needs and their feelings are of paramount importance. For us, a crying, whining, screaming, thrashing child might be just that: a child behaving undesirably. More so when according to us, they are doing so for no real reason. But for them, it is hugely important. How many times have we encountered parents who defend their ignorance of their child's needs by saying it was "nothing?" For us, it indeed might be nothing, but to them, it is as important as the world.

Being empathetic toward your child gives you the space to see the world through their eyes. It makes space for your feelings without any judgment. Empathy is the great affirmation that toddlers need that tells them, "I understand how you are feeling. It is all right. Your feelings matter to me."

Empathy lets your child feel connected to you. It gives them a sense of belonging and security. This will bring more confidence in your relationship with your child. Children who have empathetic parents are easier to manage and work with. They live with the knowledge that they have support to fall back on when they have a bad day. If the parent is always critical and lacks empathy, the child will retreat within themselves. Such parents may be unable to foster a relationship based on trust and confidence with their kids. Such children will build resentment toward their parents as time goes by. Empathy gives them the validation their feelings need.

The very first step to validation is being supported when they make mistakes. You are not accepting their behavior, rather welcoming the fact that they are humans and will make mistakes, just like you do. We are taught from our early childhood that mistakes are bad, and committing mistakes is disastrous. We are taught that making an error is akin to failure. What we need to realize is that children are innocent. They are not bad: they are pure. But when we are not welcoming of their mistakes, we are saying the exact opposite to them. When you are accusatory in your approach, kids resort to hiding and covering up their mistakes because they fear you. Hiding mistakes can never be a good idea, as one lie would need a hundred more to hide it. When you hide wrongdoings, you can neither rectify it, nor can you learn from it to avoid it in the future. Instead, be welcoming of their mistakes, guiding them gently with empathy as to how they can correct them. This is what validation gives them; a chance to get back up from their failures, learn from them, and try not to repeat them.

Validation Versus Acceptance

Many parents confuse validating their child's behavior with accepting their behavior. These are not the same thing. Validation is simply to affirm the feelings of your child as something worth taking note of. You give their feelings the respect they deserve, without brushing them off as inconsequential and meaningless. One of the biggest criticisms of the theory of empathy is that it encourages the child to feel confident about their mistakes and urges them to continue their bad behavior. This also is not true.

Validation is not equal to condoning bad behavior. You are validating the way your child feels, but not the way your child behaves. While you are empathetic toward your child, by telling them you understand their feelings and why they are angry or upset, you also firmly establish how you do not support or condone their bad behavior. See the following as an example.

A three-year-old is upset that her older brother has drank her orange juice. They get into an argument, and she throws the empty juice carton at her brother, who ducks. The empty box lands on the side table that holds crockery, knocking a glass plate to the floor, smashing it to pieces. Here, their quarrel has resulted in a broken plate and the danger of strewn glass pieces, all over the kitchen floor. Any caregiver would be angry. She was in the right by being upset, but was the ensuing argument and throwing things appropriate? How must the parent react? How would you react?

What the child needs here is for us to understand that firstly, she is only three years old. Just two years older than being an infant. Only being able to talk for one year. That is still an early age for us to be holding them to the task of proper behavior. So, what do we do? What that child needs is a hug and a rub on the back that tells them you understand. If it is a sensitive child, they would be crying, even before you look at them. A tougher child is bound to melt into your arms and cry when you give that hug. Why is this so? Because at this tender age, kids are too innocent of fostering any real animosity or negativity. Their guilt will bring those tears on. At this point, they are too overwhelmed by the loss of their juice than the loss of their own emotions. You would only be hurting them more by scolding or yelling at them.

Once they have calmed down, the crying has subsided, and they can look at you without being uncomfortable, now is the time to tell them gently it was wrong. By this time, they know that already. You have to lay down the rules when your child is calm and in a receptive enough state to listen and acknowledge what you are saying.

"I know you were upset. You were angry: your brother drank your juice. But, dearest, what just happened was not okay. You must not throw things at each other. We talk about and solve our problems. I don't want you to throw things at each other. This could have seriously hurt someone."

This much is enough to let the message sink in. But this message will only resonate in their minds when you have held them and rubbed their backs, giving them that much-needed hug. That simple, empathetic gesture broke the barrier between the parent and the child. It is what made the child more accepting of their follies and the given advice. Of course, you must not forget the older brother or his part in this whole scenario, but for now, our concentration was the vulnerable little girl of three.

Validation is like saying I get how you are feeling. I don't agree with what you did, but I understand why you did it. You can and must set behavioral limits, while being empathetic at the same time.

Strategies on How To Empathize With Your Toddler

If you are looking to be empathetic to your child's feelings, there are a few things to keep in mind to convey the right message of understanding effectively.

Bring yourself to their level. Either bend down or kneel so that you both are at the same level.

Look your child in the eye and truly listen to them. Put away any phones or electronics, or any other chore that you might be doing, to give them your undivided attention.

Reflect and repeat what they say. It is a good thing to repeat what they tell you back to them. Doing this accomplishes two things. It tells them you have understood what they are saying, and also opens up a chance to correct you if you have, in any way, misunderstood them.

Describe how they look and give them words to help them tell you how they feel. For example, you may say, "You are pounding the table with your fists; you look angry!"

Ask them appropriate questions, so you know you are understanding them correctly, validating their feelings and not the feelings you have chosen for them. For example, you might say something like, "You look sad: are you sad?" And then you let them agree or disagree.

While being empathetic, do not criticize, judge, or try to solve their problems for them. Doing this would only defeat the purpose of being empathetic in the first place.

Do not tell them: "You are feeling sad, so this is what you need . . ."

Do not tell them: "Stop crying. If you keep crying, everyone will think you are a cry baby."

Do not tell them: "You are always upset at the table during dinner."

Validating your child's feelings is just as important as teaching them manners and ethics. For toddler years, this is even more important, as at this tender age, they are unaware of the complex emotions a human being is capable of feeling, and all that they undergo is bound to be overwhelming for an innocent mind. This age needs the most amount of validation and empathy, to help the child learn the range of their own emotions and how to handle them.

Have A Meaningful Talk

Sometimes all you need is to sit and talk. What you could do is have such a conversation at bedtime with your child. Before or after story time, you could sit with your child and talk about your day. Then ask them about theirs and simply listen. It is remarkable how much a child is willing to share when you are ready to listen. Ensure that you end your conversation on a happy note that leaves your child smiling. Be it a joke, a funny story, a funny incident from your day at the office, or anything else, let the last memory of you be a happy one for your child, as they drift off to sleep.

Having such sharing sessions is a step toward empathy. It will strengthen your relationship with your child and enrich the trust factor between you both. With time, as your child grows and starts school, this very session will come in handy. Your child will be more forthcoming and trusting of you to share their day's happening with you, every day. This ease of conversation is what any parent desires, and you can have it too, with a little empathy.

Chapter 11: Daily Life of Your Toddler: Eat, Play, Love

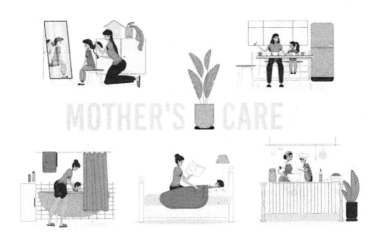

There is no doubt about it, the toddler years are a time of immense learning, growing, and development. There are so many things that our toddlers are learning daily, and parents and caregivers are responsible for providing the structure and the tools for success, as our toddlers explore their worlds, learning how to make sense of each day as it comes.

Parents and caregivers of toddlers know that each day is ripe with opportunities to guide and teach our little ones how to be successful in their daily tasks, such as eating, playing, relating to others, and sleeping. Loving and respectful discipline includes the guidance and structure that gives toddlers the tools they need to be successful in these areas.

Playtime

Playtime! For most adults, it is easy to associate playtime as time spent goofing off, or maybe even as a waste of time, but for toddlers, it is so much more. Maria Montessori, the founder, and creator of the Montessori system of schooling, famously stated that: "Play is the work of the child," and this could not be truer. What may look like a waste of time to an adult, is a toddler whose brain is rapidly developing and making new connections, as they explore, handle, and manipulate the world around them. Play is where toddlers learn how to interact with their world and everything in it. The wooden puzzle pieces they are working with offer an opportunity to develop their cognitive and problem-solving skills, to better develop their fine motor skills and their hand-eye coordination, and to experience the feeling of pride that helps to build their self-esteem, when they finally are able to place each piece in its proper place. The building block set they are using gives toddlers the opportunity to practice their fine and gross motor skills, to develop their hand-eye coordination, use their imagination, and be able to physically manipulate it into reality. They build their engineering skills, as they learn to recognize what works when building a tower and what doesn't. Shape sorters that require toddlers to place the appropriate shape through the appropriate slot encourage problem solving, spatial awareness, and perseverance, as they learn by the repetitive try-fail-try-fail-try-win model. Dolls and other figurines provide tools for toddlers to engage in the imaginative play that helps them explore and reinforce what they are learning about social dynamics and interactions. A wooden spoon and a plastic mixing bowl, turned upside down, are a drumstick and drum set that can be used to explore sound, rhythm, and beat. Toys do not need to be fancy or store-bought. They simply need to be accessible and safe.

According to the Montessori model, play is responsible for allowing children to grow socially, build their creativity muscles, and expand and strengthen their problem-solving skills, language skills, and physical skills. The Montessori model encourages open-ended toys that may be used and manipulated by children that encourage them to use their imagination to solve problems, cooperate with others, and engage their creativity. An example of open-ended toys would be toys like Lego and blocks that a toddler can choose what they want to do with.

Toddlers often make the leap from solitary play to parallel play around the age of two. Solitary play is what babies typically do, where they can fixate on an object of interest alone, by themselves for large periods of time, without needing anyone else to interact with or engage with them. Toddlers and older children will still engage in solitary play, but toddlers make the shift to parallel play, which is where they will play alongside their peers, but not in a way that appears that they are necessarily interacting together. They may be playing with similar toys or completely different toys, but they are playing side by side and enjoying the company of another child nearby. Group play does not typically develop until around the age of three. Then children are ready to being playing cooperatively and interactively, sharing, and taking turns. Before then, toddlers may appear to be uninterested in playing together, but parallel play, side by side, still offers social advantages for them at that time. All of these forms of play are useful and healthy, and toddlers should always be allowed to pursue the form of play they are authentically drawn to at the time, without being pushed into another by parents and caregivers.

As each of these forms of play has its place, the most important aspect in each is that children should be allowed to develop their own play themes. Toddlers do not need their parents and caregivers to tell or show them how to play. They simply need to be provided with a safe and accessible space to explore safe and interesting toys. In fact, this is a part of the loving and respectful guidance that allows them autonomy and choice, in a safe situation.

Routine and Rest

With great routine, comes great rest! As with the rest of their days, toddlers thrive on a predictable sleep schedule. To begin, let us look at some of the toddler sleep guidelines that have been given by the American Academy of Sleep Medicine that have been endorsed by the American Academy of Pediatrics. The American Academy of Sleep Medicine recommends that children between one and two years old should sleep between eleven and fourteen hours per day (including their naps), and that children between three and five should sleep between ten to thirteen hours per day (including their naps). The American Academy of Sleep Medicine also gives several advantages to ensuring that our children get an adequate amount of daily sleep, including improved behavior, learning, memory, attention, emotional regulation, and mental and physical health! That is more than enough to inspire parents and caregivers to ensure their toddlers are getting enough sleep, is not it?

Now the question remains, how? Most parents and caregivers have experienced one or two hiccups related to sleep and their toddler, often including falling asleep, and then staying asleep. It may be helpful to first ensure that parents and caregivers are viewing the process as a facilitator of helping their toddlers to get the kind of restorative and restful sleep that is so crucial during this period of intense growth and development, and also as a guide for future healthy sleep habits. This is a part of creating a firm foundation for the rest of their lives. Just as with so many of the other areas that parents and caregivers are tasked with guiding and teaching toddlers to be successful in, restful sleep is something in which that toddlers often blossom, with the right mindset from the people they look to for guidance. This is an area that all too often results in a struggle, as parents and caregivers find themselves focused on forcing an outcome, rather than helping their toddlers develop healthy habits that will set them on a path to success.

In order to meet the daily suggested sleep guideline, set by the American Academy of Sleep Medicine, toddlers require at least one nap during their day. Many toddlers naturally wake early sometime between six and eight in the morning. It is common for a child to take their first nap just a few hours after waking up, and this can be as long as two hours long. Many toddlers then get sleepy in the afternoon, and are ready for a mid-afternoon nap in the two to four o'clock range, and how late parents and caregivers allow for this nap to continue, will directly affect bedtime.

Common bedtimes for toddlers are typically in the window of time between six and eight o'clock. A toddler whose afternoon nap comes closer to the two o'clock time frame, will likely be ready for bed closer to six o'clock, but the toddler whose afternoon nap falls closer to the four o'clock range, will not likely be ready for bed until closer to the eight o'clock time frame.

All of these time frames and ranges are estimates, and every child and every family is different. As far as the exact times that will work for you, that will have to be figured out when examining family schedules. The first step in figuring out which sleep schedules will work best for your family is in determining when is the ideal time for your toddler to wake, and when is the ideal time for your toddler to go to sleep at night. Once you have these two times, you can work to structure naps within that time frame.

Parents and caregivers following Attachment Parenting principles will likely stay with their toddler as they are drifting off to sleep, perhaps patting them on the back, singing lullabies, telling stories in a low, calm voice, or even just snuggling into them and allowing them to drift off to sleep by their side.

Toddlers and Tech

Toddlers and tech have been a significant part of the parenting conversation since portable technology use has skyrocketed in recent years. Among toddlers who use hand-held mobile tech devices, the more time spent with these tech devices, the more likely to have delayed speech skills. In fact, a recent study showed that for every thirty-minute increase of screen time, there was a forty-nine percent increase in risk in expressive speech delay!

There is different concern, as well. Sitting down and watching a TV show in the family room is a passive activity, and any activity that encourages a child to slow down their physical movement, their cognitive engagement, and their creativity, is best to only allow in moderation. Interacting with tech through hand-held devices, such as tablets, carries additional risk by means of the sheer nature of the product. Hand-held tech devices go everywhere with us, and are often used to placate and distract toddlers in scenarios, such as waiting rooms, restaurants, and in their car seats. This is leading to a generation of children that are not developing important life skills, such as patience. There is a need for toddlers to be able to interact with the world around them. There have also been connections drawn between dwindling attention spans and heavy tech use in children.

As with all new things—and this hand-held, heavy tech use by young children is still fairly new—it is usually wise to have caution. In guiding and teaching our toddlers in a loving and respectful way, it is important to directly engage with them as we help them to build important skills such as patience, waiting for their turn, and interacting socially, as opposed to handing them distraction with a screen.

Chapter 12:   Encouraging Learning Through Sports and Books

Sports with Learning

As children begin creating, their natural abilities start to show, and they are drawn towards specific exercises. Numerous children begin utilizing sports and extracurricular exercises to make progress.

You can likewise discover increasingly extraordinary exhortation on this point, in specialists' digital recordings on the advantages of sports and exercise for children and the various sorts of sports for them.

The medical advantages of sports and games: Studies have uncovered that kids who play sports are less worried than their peers who do not partake in any physical activity. Participation in sports has numerous different advantages like expanded cardiovascular wellness, a solid development in their ligaments, bones, tendons, and muscles. They will grow better equalization and coordination and have better sleep.

There are likewise social advantages of sports for children: It encourages them to have more companions. When they join a neighborhood football or a cricket crew, or take part in school sports, it is useful to them, as they find some good competitive allies. This will likewise open the channels for an altogether new friend network for them.

It gets them outside: Many children are extremely content to remain inside, sitting in front of the TV and playing PC games; they have no inclination for genuine interaction in the external world, or to get some fresh air. At the point when they take up a sport, it is an opportunity for enjoyment, to go outside, practice building skills, and take in some sunshine. It makes a difference if they get themselves and their garments filthy. There are always great laundry products at home to deal with the stains: Surf exceeds expectations will never let you down.

They fabricate fearlessness: Sports are a decent medium to help up your youngster's confidence and improve their self-assurance. It likewise teaches them collaboration, objective structure, and accomplishment for their everyday life. And keeping in mind that by playing, on the off chance that they slip and fall, it lets them discover a workable pace for themselves.

Books with Behavior Learning

A newborn child will not comprehend most of what you are doing or why. In any case, reading to your infant is a brilliant and mutually beneficial action that you can continue for years to come, and it is significant for your infant's cerebrum.

Reading out loud:

- Teaches an infant about correspondence
- Introduces ideas, for example, numbers, letters, hues, and shapes in an enjoyable way
- Builds tuning in, memory, and jargon aptitudes

- Gives babies data about their general surroundings

When children have matured to their first birthday, they will have taken in all the sounds expected to communicate in their local language. The more stories you read, the more words your infant will have heard, and speech will come easier to them.

Hearing words assists with building a rich system of words in an infant's cerebrum. Toddlers whose parents talk and read to them frequently realize a larger number of words by the age of two than ones who have not been read to. What is more, kids who are exposed to reading during their initial years are bound to master reading at the correct time.

When you read to your infant:

- Your child hears you utilizing a wide range of feelings and expressive sounds. This enables social improvement, and enthusiastic communication.
- It urges your infant to look, point, and answer questions. This assists with social improvement and thinking aptitudes.
- Your infant improves language abilities by duplicating sounds, perceiving pictures, and learning words.

In any case, maybe the most resoundingly and significant motivation to read is that it makes an association between the things your infant cherishes the most—your voice, closeness to you, and books. Investing energy reading to your infant shows that reading is significant. What is more, if newborn children and toddlers are read to frequently with delight, fervor, and closeness, they start to connect books with joy, and new readers are made.

Various Ages, Different Stages

Young babies may not realize what the photos in a book mean, however they can concentrate on them, particularly faces, splendid hues, and various examples. When you read or sing bedtime songs and nursery rhymes, you will engage with and calm your newborn child.

Between 4–6 months:

Your infant may start to show more enthusiasm for books. Your little one will get and hold onto the books, yet will mouth, bite, and also drop them. Pick strong vinyl or material books with brilliant hues and also commonplace, dull, or rhyming content for variety.

Between 6 months–one year:

Your infant begins to comprehend that photos speak about objects, and may begin to show that they like certain photos, pages, or even whole stories more than other ones. Your child will react while you read, reaching for the book, and making sounds. By a year, your little one will turn pages (with some assistance from you), pat, or begin to understand questions on a page and rehash your sounds.

When and How to Read

Here is an incredible thing about reading out loud: it does not take unique abilities or hardware, just you, your infant, and a few books. Read for a couple of moments, but do it frequently. Try not to stress over completing whole books—center around pages that you and your child appreciate.

Attempt to read each day, maybe before nap time and bed time: reading before bed allows you and your infant to snuggle and interact. It additionally sets a normal practice that will help calm your infant.

It is additionally acceptable to read at different points in the day. Pick times when your child is dry, taken care of, and alert. Books additionally prove to be useful when you are stuck waiting, so have some in the diaper sack to occupy time sitting at the specialist's office or in line at the market.

Here are some other understanding tips:

- Cuddling while you read enables your infant to have a sense of security and warmth that is associated with you.
- Read with articulation, make your voice sequential where it is proper, or utilize various voices for various characters.
- Do not stress over after the content precisely. Stop now and again and pose inquiries or offer remarks on the photos or content. ("Where's the kitty? There he is! What a charming dark kitty.") Your kid probably will not have the option to react yet, yet this lays the preparation for doing so later.
- Sing nursery rhymes, make clever creature sounds or ricochet your infant on your knee—anything that shows that reading is entertaining.

- Babies love and gain from redundancy, so do not fear to read the same books, over and over. When you do, rehash a similar accentuation each time as you would with a commonplace melody.

As your infant gets more established, urge your little one to touch the book or hold sturdier vinyl, fabric, or board books. You would prefer not to support biting on books, however by placing them in the mouth, your child is finding out about them, discovering how books feel and taste and finding that you cannot eat them!

What to Read

Books for infants ought to have basic, monotonous, and commonplace content and clear pictures. During the initial few months of life, your youngster just prefers to hear your voice. So, you can read nearly anything, particularly books with a sing-tune or rhyming content. As your child gets progressively keen on seeing things, pick books with basic pictures with sturdy pages.

As your child gets older, you can acquire vinyl or fabric books that have faces, brilliant hues, and shapes. At the point when your infant starts to react to what is inside the books, include board books with pictures of children or well-known items like toys. When your child begins to do things like sit up in the bath or eat finger nourishments, discover basic tales about everyday schedules, like sleep time or bath time. As your child begins to talk, pick books that let babies rehash basic words or expressions.

Books with mirrors and various surfaces (crimped, delicate, and scratchy) are additionally incredible for this age group. So are crease out books you can prop up, or books with folds that pop open for a shock. Board books make page-turning simpler for newborns, and vinyl or fabric books can go all over —even the tub. Children of all ages like photograph collections with pictures of individuals they know and love. Furthermore, babies love nursery rhymes!

Probably the most ideal approaches to ensure that your little one grows up to be a reader are to have books around your home. If your infant is mature enough to slither over to a container of toys and choose one, ensure a few books are in the blend.

Other than the books you possess, you likewise can acquire some from the library. Numerous libraries possess story books for babies as well. Remember to get a book for yourself while you are there.

Chapter 13: Foods To Eat To Help Toddlers Grow Up Healthy

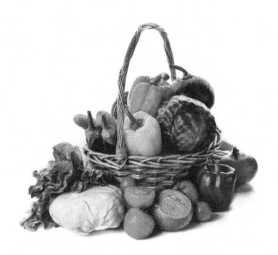

Nutrition and nurturing are deeply intertwined. Feeding a baby is a source of deep pleasure for most parents—snuggling to breastfeed, offering a warm bottle as you rock in a chair, those cute little baby food jars, the eager, O-shaped mouth awaiting the next spoonful of brightly colored mush, the first messy graham-cracker smile.

Toddlerhood brings plenty of changes to mealtimes, including more food choices, the advent of self-feeding, and newly defined tastes and opinions. It is little wonder, in the face of developments like these, that your onetime pleasure over the primal act of feeding may ripen into worry, frustration, and the occasional standoff. In fact, more feeding problems are thought to begin during the second year of life than at any other point in childhood.

The first question most parents have, once their child's food intake is no longer easily measured in bottles and jars, is how much is enough? The answer is less than you may think. The first year of life was one big growth spurt. Your child nearly tripled their birth weight in their first twelve months—gaining about a pound a month—and doubled in height. But the pace of growth drops off now, and so, correspondingly, does a toddler's appetite. What should a toddler eat?

A balanced diet can be elusive at this age. If you have a hearty, curious eater, who welcomes whatever you set before him, thank your lucky stars. Most toddlers' appetites are more whimsical. Your child may insist on a cheese sandwich, every day for lunch and dinner, for weeks at a time. They may refuse all fruits. They may devour something one day and sneer at it the next. They may go through a growth spurt and eat like a lumberjack, then seem to live on air for the next few weeks. These tendencies have little to do with your own modeling—even gourmands have kids who eat nothing but American cheese on white bread. Relax. Studies show that if they are offered a healthful variety of foods, toddlers have a remarkable innate ability to self-select just what and how much they need to survive.

In fact, their total intake may veer from a few hundred calories at one meal to as many as a thousand at the next. What your child consumes over the course of a week or two is more important than the nutrient breakdown of a single meal, or a single day's meals. The right balance averages out on its own. What follows is a description of a toddler's overall nutritional needs, in very general terms. Keep in mind that the typical toddler serving is much smaller than that of an adult. The rule of thumb is that a serving equal about one tablespoon of each food per year of age (that works out to one tablespoon for a twelve-month-old, two and a half tablespoons for a thirty-month-old).

Dairy. No more than twenty-four ounces of milk in twenty-four hours, or about two to three cups per day, for eight hundred total milligrams of calcium per day. Most children switch to whole milk (from breast milk or formula) at twelve months of age, or begin to supplement breast milk with whole milk. By age two, your pediatrician may advise a switch to milk with a lower fat content, but do not it unless you are so advised, as this recommendation depends on the individual child's overall health and diet. Remember that calcium is found in cheese, yogurt, and ice cream as well. Some toddlers can be cajoled to drink milk to which a little chocolate syrup has been added—not harmful in small amounts. Pediatricians recommend that toddlers' milk not be served in a bottle, to prevent overfeeding.

Proteins. Two to three servings per day in the first year, then four to five servings. Options include meats, fish, eggs, cheese, tofu, and beans. A serving may be less than one-fourth of an adult-sized portion, or about one ounce.

Fruits and vegetables. Three to five servings a day. Remember that fruits and vegetables can be mixed into other foods too (such as berries in muffins or grated zucchini in spaghetti sauce). Limit juice to eight ounces per day (which can be diluted). Any one hundred percent juice is fine, but do not rely on juice alone for this food group. Whole fruits and vegetables provide added fiber and vitamins. Note that some orange juice brands have added calcium, helpful if your child dislikes milk or cheese.

Grains. Three servings daily in the first year, then four servings. Includes breads, hot or cold cereals, teething biscuits, crackers, rice, and pasta. Serve healthier one hundred percent whole-wheat products as much as possible to orient your child's taste to them.

Fats. Roughly ten percent of the daily total. Includes butter, oils, and peanut butter. (Spread peanut butter thinly, as it can be a choking hazard. It is not recommended for ages under two.) Most of these foods should be chopped, mashed, or pureed versions of what the rest of the family eats. You may also use stage-three baby foods, although as they get more teeth, many older babies suddenly rebel against anything they cannot pick up themselves, which means the mushy stuff is out.

It is useful to keep on hand a few jars of the toddler-style baby foods. Their textures are like adult foods and provide variety in a pinch. Should you give your child a daily vitamin? That is a call for your pediatrician to make. In general, it may not be necessary if your child enjoys a wide variety of foods and is a good eater. If, like many toddlers, however, your child is finicky, goes on food jags, or refuses a food group (such as vegetables, fruit, or milk) altogether, a multivitamin can provide a nutritional safety net. Select a brand formulated for children. A younger toddler needs liquid vitamins. After about eighteen months (depending on how many teeth your child has), a chewable children's vitamin may be prescribed. In addition to having the proper nutritional composition, fun colors, flavors, and shapes ensure they will be eaten. Because they can look like candy, however, avoid poisonings from overconsumption by storing all vitamins out of reach of children.

Smart Mealtime Routines

In theory, things are supposed to get simpler now that your child can help feed himself. Yet fretting over food is a leading concern that parents bring to their pediatricians during their child's second and third years of life. Why the disparity? Because parents, in their concern about rearing a healthy child, tend to fixate on this very visible, controllable part of life. Keep telling yourself: my toddler will not starve or suffer malnutrition. Let his own natural appetite be his feeding guide. If you focus on making eating pleasant and avoid power struggles, everything else should be, well, a piece of cake. Here are the golden rules of feeding toddlers:

Feed them when they are hungry. If It is close to a meal, give them a quick, nutritious snack—such as a piece of bread or a bowl of applesauce—to tide them over until everyone sits down together. Exception: if your child is continually hungry just twenty or thirty minutes after a meal has ended, they are not eating enough at meals and may be relying on snacks too much. Try making them wait until the next set snack-time or meal to curb the habit.

Introduce the idea of regular feeding times. You should not ignore a toddler who is spiraling out of control because their little tummy is howling with hunger. At the same time, for your own sanity and for your child's benefit, establish a feeding schedule of three meals and two or three snacks, all at about the same time every day. Eating on a predictable schedule helps pace a toddler's energy and underscores a sense of security. A child is also more likely to eat well at meals and try new foods if they have not been snacking all day. For safety's sake, serve food at the table or highchair. This also prevents the habit of your child noshing while doing something else.

Do not isolate them. Although your child's small tummy may not be in sync with the rest of the family's, that is no excuse for serving them all their meals segregated from everyone else. They should be seated with the family for breakfast, lunch, and dinner. Even if they have had his meal earlier, let them have dessert or a snack while everyone else eats. By dining together, you are modeling a healthy attitude toward a variety of foods, as well as basic table manners.

Keep portions small. Little bits at a time are more appealing for a child, not to mention less messy for you. If your child wants seconds, let them ask for it. Never demand that your child join the "clean-plate club" (to which you may have belonged as a youngster). Also outdated: cutesy here-comes-the-airplane gimmicks. They might work to get an easily distracted diner to finish a few more bites, but once they are signaling that they are full, do not force more. Cajoling by handfeeding is also time-consuming for you and does not promote self-feeding. Nor should you restrict portions. By only giving your child "this much and no more," you risk fueling an insecurity about having enough to eat, which can backfire into overeating. Unsure when they will get to fill up again, the child begins to stuff themselves whenever the opportunity for unrestricted dining presents itself. Left to their own devices, toddlers are naturally able to stop when they are full, even in the middle of dessert.

Do not push, but do not stop trying, either. If your child turns up her nose at a new food, do not give up on it. Serve it again a week later. Some toddlers must see a food two dozen times or more before it becomes familiar enough to be acceptable. (The opposite is true too: sometimes a well-liked food inexplicably loses favor.) Realize, too, that some children are more generally averse to all things new. At a later meal, offer another tiny portion of it. The food may have grown strange because the child has not seen it in a while, or it could just be a phase. Vegetable hating—the sudden dislike of anything green or orange that grows in the ground— commonly sprouts up at age two and can last for several years. Do not insist. Just keep serving them in a low-key way. Be prepared to admit temporary failure.

Do not use food as a reward. Many parents swear by M&M candies as incentives for potty training. Or they promise checkout-line candy at the grocery store, if the child behaves well during a shopping excursion. The treat is well-intentioned and the effect, at least in the short term, may be great. But by using food as a reward or bribe, you are setting up an association with food as a source of comfort, praise, and love. A better choice is to offer treats "just because."

Chapter 14: How to Raise Autonomous and Cooperative Children

Raising children to be independent persons separate from Mom and Dad is one of the most important tasks of parenting. When we allow children to do things for themselves, deal with their own problems, and learn from their own mistakes, we enable them to develop their own values and arm them with self-reliance and confidence in their own capacities, both of which they will need as they navigate the world on their own.

But what does this have to do with discipline? Think about it. When people are placed in positions where they are dependent, they inevitably have to deal with massive feelings of helplessness, resentment, worthlessness, anger, frustration, inferiority, and embarrassment. As sad as it sounds, this happens with parents and their offspring as well. When our children are small, their age and inexperience make them wholly dependent on us; but as they grow, their dependency can lead to hostility, and we then have to deal with issues of discipline, disrespect, and rebelliousness, usually during the teen years. To avoid this, we have to teach them, show them, and tell them what they need to learn about the world, while minimizing their feelings of dependency.

Follow these tips for encouraging autonomy:

1. Allow children to make some choices for themselves.
2. Gabrielle wants to wear leopard print leggings with a rainbow-colored tutu, a neon pink top, apple green rain boots, glittery fairy wings, a tiara, and forty-

seven different plastic bracelets to a field trip. You think she looks like a walking mini circus, but you let her wear the entire outfit anyway. Why? Decisions about clothing choices might seem inconsequential in the grand scheme of things, but to children, each small choice they get to make is one more opportunity to take some control of their own lives. Especially when they are young, there is so much about their lives that are beyond their control. Allowing them to decide on the little things is the first step to autonomy. However, there are occasions when instead of handing over the reins, it is better to offer the child a choice about how something can be done. For instance, if little Madeleine refuses to take her medicine, you cannot simply say, "Ok, that's fine. Have it your way." Instead, try saying something like, "I know you do not like how this tastes. How about mixing a bit of apple juice with it to make it yummy?"

3. Stop asking questions all day long.

4. "Did you have fun today?" "How did you like it?" "What did you do?" "Was Agnes there?" "Where are you, Stella? What are you doing?" Questions, questions, questions. All day long. Never-ending and intrusive. Of course, It is perfectly fine to ask your child about his day and how he is, but bombarding children with questions often causes them to clam up instead of opening to you. And worse, even when you are really just asking out of curiosity, to a child, the question "Did you have fun?" can seem loaded.

Imagine if the child actually had an awful time, and now, they have to tell you about it, which would then make you feel disappointed—on top of his own disappointment. Often, the best way to figure out what is going on with our children and to get them to engage with us is to just listen. This way, they get to form their own opinions and feelings about the goings-on in their world. They get to freely share what they think and how they feel, without worrying about your judgment.

5. Stop answering questions all day long.

6. When a child asks you a question, do not rush to answer it. You are doing her a disservice if you do. Usually, before a child asks a question ("How do fountains work?" "What kind of tree is a Groot?" "Who made God?"), he or she has already given the question some thought. Small children ask questions, not because they need a definitive answer, but because they need a sounding board to help them further explore their questions and take their thinking processes further. When you give a child an immediate, "correct" answer, you stop the thought process. Instead of giving a child an answer, what actually helps them and encourages autonomous thinking is to parry with another question that will further their exploration of the topic at hand.

7. Acknowledge that children struggle.

8. When you introduce a task by telling a child that it is easy, you are setting them up to fail. If they succeed

in doing it, there is no gratifying sense of accomplishment. It was easy anyway. If they fail, then they have failed at something easy. This is very embarrassing and disheartening. On the other hand, if you say something like, "This can be a little tough," or "It is not easy, but go ahead and try," you give the child different parameters to work with. If they succeed, there is a great feeling of having accomplished something difficult. If they fail, they, at least, fail with the recognition that they attempted to do something hard. We, as parents, often think that it is best to push children into doing tasks that will teach them to be independent. To test them. To toughen them up. We often forget that some tasks are hard for children, especially when they are doing it for the first time. In the process of raising independent, able young people, we also need to respect their struggles and not push them too hard.

9. Encourage children to look for answers and resources outside the home.

10. One of the best ways to reduce children's feelings of dependency on the family, is to introduce resources outside the home and to encourage children to make good use of these resources. Teach your child that the world is filled with numerous people, places, services, opportunities, and experiences to guide them in their journey. All of these are just waiting to be discovered. The world is not a scary place. They will get help when they need it if they know where to

look. This is a valuable lesson and it is great in one more way: it reduces the pressure on the parents to be experts on everything, to have all the answers. Put children in situations where they can learn from others. Let Grandma teach the little ones about fruits and vegetables as they care for her garden. Let the doctor explain how a diet made up mostly of sugary foods wreaks havoc on the body. Let the science whiz at the office assist your young learner with his school project. Parents are, of course, their children's first (and, possibly, best) teachers. But as children grow, there are places outside the home where children will learn more about specific topics than they ever could from Mom or Dad.

11. Encourage children to dream.

12. As parents, we think it just and prudent to prepare children for the worst. We do not want them to be disappointed. We want them to be realistic. We do not want their heads perpetually stuck in the clouds. When Ella asks if Mom and Dad would agree to turning the house into a castle fit for a princess, Dad laughs, and Mom says, "Of course not! Do not be silly." Here is the thing: never, ever take away a child's hope. Even as an adult, you might agree that one of the pleasures of life is the dreaming, the wishing, the fantasizing. Even more so for children. Little ones live in a world filled with endless possibilities. When we try to guard them against the possibility of disappointment, we often rob them of

important, life-enriching experiences. So, the next time Ava asks if you can buy her a pony, do not bring her reveries to a screeching halt by saying, "We do not have the money for that!" Instead of telling her that it is out of the question, engage her in conversation about her love for ponies. You might try saying, "Are not ponies great? What do you think they eat? Do you think they like apples?" Often, children are not as concerned about the actual having something, as they are about exploring the idea of "what if?"

We can engage our children's cooperation without making them feel bad about themselves or ruining their self-esteem. The rules below are simple enough to follow, and they will help you raise cooperative children in a respectful and loving environment.

1. Limit what you say.
2. There is really no need to be sarcastic, to name-call, or to use any of the tactics we enumerated above. Communicating with children can be as simple as just describing what is there. "There are clothes on the floor. They need to be picked up," instead of "Why are you such a slob? Clean up this room!" "The juice spilled. We need a kitchen towel," instead of "Cannot you drink juice without getting it all over yourself? Ugh!" Using the word "you" can come off accusatory, and may lead to children getting defensive, so drop it. Instead of "You broke the mug.

Sweep it up," try saying, "The mug broke. We need a broom here."

3. One word is often enough.

4. Parents are often surprised to find out how well this works. When you use one-word statements, interactions with children are easier and take less time. You avoid long-winded explanations and making your children feel oppressed by your commands. When a thirteen-year-old hears his parent say, "Lawn" or "Light" or "Coat," he gets an opportunity to figure out what needs to be done and to work from his own initiative. "Oh, I forgot to mow the lawn. I'll do it now." Take care, though, that you not use your child's name as the one word. When Anna hears her name in a stern or disapproving tone, numerous times a day, she may learn to associate it with reproach.

5. Offer some explanation.

6. We can avoid repeats of unfortunate incidents, if we take the time to give a little more information that children can use for the rest of their lives. "When you squeeze the bottle too hard, you get ketchup all over your plate." "When you do not put food back in the fridge, it can go bad." "When you disturb people while they're sleeping, they can get really mad at you." Leave out whatever sarcasm, insult, or threat you used to add at the end. Instead of saying: "Wipe your shoes on the mat before you come in, Jeff! I've

told you a million times!" stick to: "When you do not wipe your shoes, you track mud all over the house."

7. Let them know how you feel.

8. Do not worry, children can handle it. Instead of lashing out at your child because you are too tired to deal with whatever he is asking of you, accept what you are feeling and let him know what is going on. "Tony, this is not a good time. I am tired, and I need to lie down for a while. After my nap, we'll go through your project." Doing this is a good way to avoid tension and it teaches children that adults struggle, just like them.

Chapter 15:   Building Self-Belief in Your Child

Your child's self-esteem greatly influences their learning and social behavior. If your child has low self-esteem, he or she is less likely to take risks, get out of their comfort zone and try out new experiences. On the other hand, a child with high self-esteem tends to take risks in life, makes friends faster and succeed in school. Basically, having self-esteem is the key to your child's mental wellness and social happiness. It is not only important during childhood, but also in the future as an adult. Can you think of a time in your life when you were feeling sad, and another moment when you were happy and carefree? Wasn't it much easier to relate to other people in the second scenario than in the first one?

This is what self-esteem can do to your child. Self-esteem can be defined simply as essentially what your child sees when they look in the mirror. Simply put, how they like the person they see. You need to make your child look inside himself or herself and feel comfortable with who they are. Let them believe that this self is someone who is worthy of love and one who can make things happen. Some of the behavioral problems in children are caused by a low self-image both in parents and children. Why is it delightful to be in the company of one person and a total nightmare being in the company of another? How you value yourself, perform in school, get along with others, succeed in work, and manage your marriage, all depends on the strength of your self-image. However, having a high self-worth does not mean being arrogant or narcissistic; it simply means having a real sense of understanding of your strengths and weaknesses, rejoicing in the strengths and working on the weaknesses.

Your duty as a parent is to ensure that no matter how much negative setbacks your child will encounter, they will be able to overcome them with the positive influence builders that you will instill in them.

How to Develop Healthy Self Esteem In Your Child?

In order to build your child's self-esteem, the first thing you need to do is to concentrate on their strengths and determine their areas of expertise. In addition, you need to set realistic responsibility by developing in them self-help skills when they are young. Help them to develop courage and confidence in being imperfect, and acknowledge mistakes as a part of learning. Let them have the attitude that everything and anything is possible. You can even establish a star chart or achievement board to record their successes, and look for small achievements and victories to celebrate them. However, do not forget; never compare your kids, other than only to themselves. This is the first parenting skill that you should learn; but it is never too late.

Your child's self-esteem fluctuates as they grow and is affected by their life experiences and perceptions. As such, you need to distinguish between healthy and unhealthy self-esteem in your child. The most evident characteristic of a child with a low self-esteem and/or self-worth is that they tend to have negative thoughts and say negative things about themselves. They give in easily, have a low frustration tolerance level, and tend to wait for someone else to take action, even when they end up being disappointed in themselves. On the other hand, a child with a healthy self-esteem normally enjoys interacting with others, is comfortable in social settings, and loves participating in group activities. So, what can you do if you notice that your child has a low self-esteem? Here are a few ideas:

Mind your words.

Kids tend to be oversensitive to what you as a parent, and others say. Always praise them even when they have not succeeded, both for the job well done and their effort. For instance, instead of saying, "Too bad you couldn't make the soccer team," you could instead say, "Sorry, you didn't make the soccer team, but am very proud you put so much effort into it." You might find that they do not have that particular skill or talent, so if you help them overcome that disappointment, it can help them learn what they are actually good at and develop those skills. Use humor and warmth to make them feel good about themselves, and appreciate and learn what makes them special.

Be a good role model

Being pessimistic, unrealistically harsh on yourself, or unsure about your limitations and abilities can rub off on your children. Develop your own self-worth and self-esteem, to help you grow to become a great role model that your kids can emulate.

Recognize and vent inaccurate beliefs

It is your responsibility, as a parent, to identify what your kids irrationally believe about themselves be it perfection, ability, attractiveness, or anything else. If you help them achieve higher standards and evaluate themselves more realistically, it will help them develop a healthier self-image. Inaccurate beliefs about self can settle in eventually and become a reality to them. For instance, a child who finds math challenging but performs well in school could say, "I'm not good at math and thus I'm a poor student." This is not only a false generalization, but also a belief that can prove to be an ingredient for failure. Encourage your kid to see every situation in a more positive way. A great response could be: "You are a great student, and do well in school. You only need to spend more time on math. We can work on it together."

Be affectionate and spontaneous

Being affectionate and loving can help improve your child's self-esteem. Give your kids hugs and tell them you are proud of them, when you see them trying out something new or an activity that they failed previously. Stick their lunchboxes with such messages as: "I think you are awesome!" Praise them honestly and frequently, but do not overdo it. Children with an inflated self-esteem can start to put others down, or feel that they are better than other people.

Give an accurate and positive feedback

Avoid giving out comments that might make your kid feel like they can't control their outbursts. In contrast, you could tell them that you appreciate the fact that they were angry with their sibling, but it was nice that they were able to talk it out rather than hitting or yelling. This makes them feel that you appreciate their feelings, that their choice has been rewarded, and encourages them to make the same right choice next time.

Create a secure and loving environment

Raising a child in an unsafe environment, or where they are frequently abused can greatly lower their self-esteem, more so if the parents fight and argue frequently. This can make your child feel like they have no control over their environment, which can lead to depression and a feeling of helplessness. Make sure that you also look out for signs of problems at school, abuse by others, difficulty with peers, and other contributing factors that can affect their self-esteem. Encourage them to communicate with you, or other adults that you trust, about big problems that may prove too difficult for them to solve on their own.

Encourage your kids to participate in constructive experiences

Involvement in certain activities that discourage competition and promote cooperation can be especially helpful in boosting self-esteem. Mentoring programs, for instance, where the younger child is assisted by an older one in learning, can work wonders for children. Volunteering and participating in your local community can also help with self-esteem.

When encouraging positive self-esteem, you don't want your kid to have too much or too little. It is important that they don't feel like being normal or average means that they are not good enough or are not special.

Chapter 16:   9 Common Discipline Mistakes Even Great Parents Make

Disciplining your toddlers alone is not enough. You must also avoid the common pitfalls of parenting. Many of these blunders do not just decrease the effectiveness of the discipline that you impose on your toddler but may even encourage your toddlers to misbehave. Here are the common mistakes that many parents make when disciplining their children.

1. Being Aggressive

Some parents simply give up and become aggressive. The problem with being aggressive is that the children learn nothing except fear. They do not get to understand the value that you want them to learn. Instead, they obey you out of fear. Studies also show that toddlers who have experienced aggressive or abusive parents are likely to grow aggressive as well. Being aggressive does not just mean spanking your kids, but it also includes using highly offensive words and threatening words. It is important to note that you are dealing with a toddler and being aggressive is the worst thing you can do.

2. Comparing Yourself with Other Parents

Stop comparing yourself with other parents. How they discipline their kids is their problem. If one of your friends tells you that slapping your kid in the face is effective, even if he could prove it, do not follow the advice right away. After all, according to various studies, slapping or hitting your kids is not really an effective way to discipline them.

3. Comparing Your Child with Other Children

It is wrong to compare your child with other children, except if it will be something that will make him feel good about himself. Would you like your child to compare you in terms of money with a parent who is much richer than you are? Of course not. In the same way, you should not compare your child with other children. Your toddler is unique in his own way, and you should appreciate him as he is.

4. Lying

Some parents lie to their toddlers to make them obey. Although this may work from time to time, it also has bad consequences. In a case study of a mom from New Jersey with a two-year-old daughter, it so happened that one day, when her child did not want to get in the car, she pointed at her neighbor's house nearby and told her child that it was a daycare center full of cavemen from a scary TV show. She told her daughter that she had two choices, to get in the car or be left alone in the house with a threat of being attacked by creepy cavemen. Of course, her daughter finally gave in and entered the car. Now, if you look at what happened, it would seem that it was successful. There was no shouting or spanking or anything that took place. However, the problem here occurred after the incident. Following the case study, the mom's daughter began to have a fear of daycare centers, thinking that such places have scary cavemen. As you can see, although the mother was able to make her child get into the car, the consequence was worse. Therefore, instead of lying, the best way is to be honest and be emphatic.

5. Thinking That You Understand Your Toddler

The truth is that you cannot always understand your toddler. This is simply because toddlers do not think the same way as adults do. You simply cannot tell exactly how certain things have an impact on your toddler's feelings and thoughts. More importantly, you do not know just up to what degree. Therefore, do not be too hard on your toddler.

6. Raising the Child You Want

Do not impose your life or your will upon your toddler. Your child has his own life. Let him pursue whatever he wants. Let him paint his own dreams and believe in them. Focus on the child whom you already have, and not the idea of a child in your mind whom you would wish to have. Your child may not be wired the way you would want him to be, and this is normal. Let your child have his chance in life. Let him believe and live his dreams.

7. Correcting Everything at The Same Time

Many parents try to correct all the inappropriate behaviors of their child, and they expect a toddler to be able to do it within a short period of time. This is a very unreasonable expectation. Even you cannot change your bad manners and behaviors quickly, so do not expect your toddler to be able to do it, much more than you can. Not to mention, most parents complaints about their toddlers are actually normal behaviors (or misbehaviors) for a toddler.

You must learn to pick your battles, and do not even attempt to win everything at the same time. You may start with the behavior that you consider to be the most serious and requires attention. Once you have corrected it, then you can move to another. Of course, you should discipline your child with every opportunity that presents itself. But, learn to focus on a particular behavior, so you can also gauge the effectiveness of the technique or techniques that you are using.

8. Long Explanations

Long explanations do not work on toddlers. You will only seem like talking gibberish after a few minutes. Do not forget that toddlers have a short attention span; therefore, long explanations do not work well with them. For example, you do not have to lecture your toddler why eating cookies before bedtime is not good for her teeth. She will learn that when the right time comes. Instead, just say, "No cookies." You do not have to explain so much. After all, toddlers are not meant to be very logical. They do not care so much about explanations. Of course, this rule is subject to exceptions, such as when the toddler himself wants to know the reason behind something or when giving an explanation appears to be the best course of action.

9. Bribe

Do not bribe your toddler just to make them do what you want. Otherwise, they will always ask for it, which could be a problem in the long run. In a case study in Montclair, New Jersey, a mom offered her daughter a piece of chocolate so her toddler would eat her meal. Needless to say, it worked well. Her daughter finished her meal quickly. Up to this point, it would seem that bribing is also effective. However, what happened after that, was her daughter would always ask her mother to give her a piece of chocolate, so that she would finish her meal.

Instead of bribing your child, the suggested way is to help them realize the importance of food. Using the aforesaid case study, the better way would be to tell her child that she will get hungry late in the evening if she ate so little, and that she will not be healthy, which could make her sick. If you face a similar problem with your child, you can tell them about the health benefits of the food, like it could make their skin more beautiful, make her taller or smarter, and others—but do not lie.

Toddlers usually have so many questions. As a parent, you tend to answer their questions as much as you can. It is worth noting that you should not lie to your child when they ask questions. However, you can make silly answers, but be sure that they know that it is a joke when you do so. Also, avoid giving creepy answers or those that will tend to scare your child. So, avoid answers that relate to ghosts and other scary stuff. However, parents get too caught up with answering their child's countless questions that they miss another important thing to do: to ask their child questions.

If you make the time to ask your toddler questions, even crazy and illogical ones, you might just be surprised by the answers that you might hear. Toddlers have a powerful imagination and are very curious and open to almost everything. By asking questions of your child, you will also understand how they think, and even appreciate how young they truly are—so all the more reason why you should never be aggressive or harsh with your toddler.

Conclusion

Parenting children requires that parents and caregivers be mentally stable. The most important thing we do is parenting. What does nurturing really do? Good parenting involves keeping your child safe, displaying love and listening to your child, maintaining order and discipline, setting and imposing boundaries, spending time with your child, tracking interactions and behaviors with your child, and most importantly, leading by example. Your kids are going to copy everything, good or bad, that you do. Look in the mirror to see how your child looks at you.

Understanding how children connect with others, avoiding questions, and appreciating your children for who they are will go a long way in building a positive relationship with your child, even if they don't speak yet. Most people try to cultivate a healthy relationship with those around them. We all want special ties with those we care about. A positive relationship with those we care about makes our lives genuinely enriching and makes us feel safe and loved. There are a variety of things you can do to create and sustain a healthy relationship with your wife, child, parents, or friends. Above all else, try not to take anything for granted. We have no idea what tomorrow holds, but we need to make the best of what we now have, and remind everyone around us that we care for them, and we love them. For some people, that does not come naturally, but when it is too late, you can regret not taking their chance.

You need to spend some time talking to each other and listening. This is important because you have a good relationship with others. It may be as difficult as setting aside time to spend with each other, but it means a lot of sharing stories, trusting each other, and learning what is going on in the life of the other person. In particular, children want to be heard by their parents, and they need attention. When someone tries to tell you something, it is so easy to switch off, so instead of having them repeat it to you, take some time out and listen, and remember, they came to you because they trust you and in what you have to offer.

Next, you have to consider give and take. One-sided relationships never go the distance. You ought to consider the point of view of the other person: you do not necessarily have to be right. Indeed, showing you are wrong, or apologizing where you are at fault, portrays confidence and care for the relationship. Take the time to ask for their feedback on issues that matter most to you. You will not only get another insightful perspective; you will make them feel unique.

Acceptance of who they are is also crucial for building a positive relationship with others. Remember that constant criticism is quick to get you nowhere. Although some negative feedback can be supported in small doses, the relationship will only be ruined by a constantly negative situation. Know you should not accuse others; that will not build a good relationship for anybody. If things are not moving as you like them, it is not the fault of someone else. You must make life decisions, and you are accountable for the choices that you make. Blaming others for your frustrations and defaults is definitely wrong; instead, keep asking yourself, "How can I make things better?" look within yourself for the answers—until you affect the change in the situation.

Notes:

BOOK 2: ADHD PARENTING

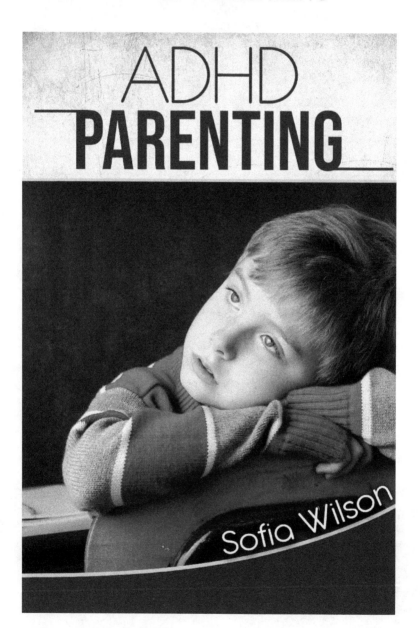

Introduction

This is meant for parents of children dealing with attention deficit / hyperactivity disorder (ADHD), whether or not they already receive treatment for their children. It will encourage you in a better way to understand ADHD and bring you with your child on a different course. You will discover new ways to prevent the development of ADHD behavior and help your child meet expectations more effectively on his own and through communicating with others.

Have you found that when participating in an event he initiates and loves, your child is much less hyperactive, impulsive and inattentive? For starters, he might be able to play for hours on end with interlocking blocks if left to himself. Time for self-directed play is very important for kids, and they may not like to have to adapt to the limits of their behavior and other activities they do. Kids may feel uncomfortable being guided or forced to act in some respects, and this anxiety makes ADHD behavior more likely. Sadly, kids need to have limitations and expectations because they have not yet understood about life's risks and needs.

So how do you describe forms that are easy for both of you to interact? How do you get your kid to agree when he tries to do something else without any trouble? How can you help him assume responsibility and autonomy slowly as he needs you to do something for him? How can you get him to follow when nobody watches over him?

You'll see when you read this that it's not all that rough. But be willing to be patient. While threats and demands can produce instant conformity, it is vastly superior to help your child learn self-reliance and cooperation, but it can take much longer. Occasionally, if your actions are effective, you may be uncertain. For instance, if your child throws a tantrum and you don't react, in the short term, you essentially allow the unwelcomed behavior. But in the long term, your unwillingness to feed into the drama can be very successful. You may also worry if you're lenient or if you're letting your kid get away with wrongdoing when you're using this new parenting style.

You might think you're incompetent or you're not doing everything you can to get out of his issues. The techniques, though, are not at all permissive. You can find that as you bring them into use, you are more assertive and stronger than you were. And the sooner you start, the earlier.

This will help make the child's behavior more mature. Finally, instead of relying on your notes, he will do more on his own.

These behaviors of parenting constitute the basis of the method, so keep them in mind.

Chapter 1: What is Attention-Deficit/Hyperactivity Disorder (ADHD)?

ADHD has long been called the "hidden" disability as the affected individuals do not look different, but do behave differently. Normal parenting methods do not work well and so ADHD can make family life quite stressful. In the classroom, the affected individual does not respond well to typical classroom management and as a result may disrupt the process of teaching. ADHD is more common than thought affecting 5.27% of all children and adolescents worldwide which translates into 1 to 2 students per class. Into adulthood 4% of adults are affected by this disorder.

This is a medical term that is given to individuals that show a persistent, developmentally inappropriate and impairing pattern in their behavior. Examples are:

- Inattention. Easily distracted and has problems paying attention

- Hyperactivity. Extensive fidgeting

- Impulsivity. Intrudes and interrupts others

A medical definition of Attention-Deficit/Hyperactivity Disorder (ADHD) is a neurobiological condition that becomes more obvious in the preschool and early years in school. A neurobiological disorder, such as ADHD, Autism and Schizophrenia, is an illness of the nervous system that is caused by genetic, biological and metabolic factors.

The 2 Clusters of Behavioral Symptoms And 3 Subtypes Of ADHD

1. Inattentive subtype, (ADD)

2. Hyperactive-Impulsive subtype

3. Combined type, (ADHD)

How Does a Child with ADHD Behave?

- More often than seems normal for their age group, he/she can get into a high state of agitation

- Is constantly moving, will often talk in a loud and incessant manner, will frequently switch from one activity to a random other without any pause

- Is incapable of filtering unimportant stimuli - everything captures their attention

- Will annoy everyone without being able to help it

- Possibly disliked by others and may realize this

- Has a low self-esteem and will often dislike him or herself?

- Shows remorse for misbehaving and will often admit to not being able to control it

- Continues on the same patterns of behavior in an enduring and persistent way

It should be noted that symptoms vary across different contexts and may also vary within the same individual's behavior from minute to minute and day to day and are different from one situation to another. There is an increase in symptoms during high cognitive demanding activities or with little active engagement. Behavior symptoms of ADHD are just the tip of the iceberg where there may be a variety of learning problems.

ADHD Symptoms – Inattention

- Struggles to concentrate

- Does not seem to listen

- Does not see a task to the end

- Demonstrates difficulty organizing work

- Avoids and will often show dislike for lengthy tasks that require effort

- Often loses things

- Easily distracted

Examples of inattention in school

Demonstrates difficulty organizing work - Disorganized desk or bag that is in disarray, papers that are shoved into the bag or miss filed.

Often loses things - Is always in want of items like pens and books and constantly hunting for them.

Easily distracted - Is always looking at what others are doing, and any noise or activity pulls the student away from the task at hand.

ADHD Symptoms — Hyperactivity/Impulsivity (At least 6 of 9 symptoms)

- Hyperactivity

- Cannot sit still, squirmy

- Struggles to play quietly

- Inappropriately leaves the seat

- Runs and climbs excessively

- Always busy

- Talks a lot and excessively

Impulsivity

- Talks without thinking and inappropriately

- Cannot wait their turn

- Often interrupts and intrudes upon others

Examples of Hyperactivity/Impulsivity in school

Always busy – Always moving whether swinging of the legs, rocks the chair or shifting in the seat.

Inappropriately leaves the seat – Has a tendency to not sit and instead wanders around and prefers to stand.

Cannot wait their turn – Shows disruptive and frustrating behavior when has to wait for his/her turn to speak and will instead interrupt by shouting out answers.

ADHD Differs in Boys and Girls

Girls are less likely to show the typical disruptive behavior symptoms that boys exhibit and for girls, they are as likely to show covert symptoms of ADHD and are as impaired academically, cognitively and socially as boys. Girls are also more likely to show verbal aggression.

Notes:

Chapter 2: How ADHD is Diagnosed

It is not very often easy to determine ADHD in a child. Your child displaying any of the symptoms described above may not be an indication that he has ADHD. Many of the actions or behaviors are really normal childhood activities. Children love to be on the move, especially when they are with others, and therefore may have the same temperament if in an environment where they are expected to keep still. In addition, if many children find that they can get away from not doing tasks, they will do anything to get out of it. It will need the constant attention and supervision of care-givers to ensure that they remain focused.

A child displaying some behavior may also be undergoing stress that may be brought on by problems being experienced at home or at school. It is therefore important that caregivers and parents are attentive to their children and notice when things are happening differently so that they can help them. As parents, you perhaps will be the first to notice any extra-ordinary behavior of your child. You have to give him too much attention to keep him focused. You have to be calling to him way too often as he seems not to be mindful of the unsafe things he does. Or, he constantly disrupts events and keeps others distracted by his actions which others do not consider well-behaved.

Sometimes as parents we may not even be aware of these behaviors, but those who are more experienced, and professionals can better discern that something is not normal in how the child functions. Also, other family members may not be so happy with the child's behavior and may consider him rude and untrained.

The pediatrician will ask questions to determine:

- How the child is doing in school.

- If your child is happy in school.

- If there are problems with learning that you or your child's teacher has observed.

- If the child has any problem completing classwork or homework.

- If there are concerns with behavior in school or when playing with friends.

The answer that you give can require that you seek to refer him to a specialist for further evaluation.

ADHD is a commonly misunderstood disorder, and therefore, everything must be done to ensure that it is properly diagnosed. This further assessment will seek to rule out other conditions that could possibly be affecting your child. Therefore, you may be asked questions to determine:

- Any learning disabilities

- Any infection of the middle ear

- Any problem hearing or seeing

- Any medical problems

- Detection of anxiety or depression or other mental problems

The specialist will also seek to consult with the child's school and caregivers on behaviors displayed. The evaluation will identify behaviors in different situations, such as when playing with friends, when playing with siblings, or in the classroom. All this is done to ensure that there is no other problem that is affecting your child. In fact, the following have to be verified before a child can be considered having ADHD:

- Symptoms appear in two or more settings, such as home and school.

- The severity of the symptoms is such that it is affecting social and educational aspects of his life.

- The child has been displaying symptoms for six months or more and before the age of 12 years.

Notes:

Chapter 3:   Causes of ADHD

Since attention deficit impulsivity disorder (ADHD) signs lack of attention, aggression, and hyperactivity impact a kid's potential to understand and even get together with many others, certain may believe that the behavior of an ADHD kid is triggered by either a lack of knowledge, a dysfunctional home environment, or perhaps too much tv. Evidence currently shows ADHD is primarily a neurological disease. Some external conditions, though, may also play a part. Here we distinguish fact from opinion about ADHD reasons.

Pesticides

Investigation suggests a possible link between pesticides and ADHD. A 2010 research in pediatricians found higher rates of ADHD in kids with higher concentrations of outside organophosphate in the urine, an insecticide utilized on goods.

Another study in 2010, had shown that people with a higher concentration of organophosphate in urine were much more probable to have a kid with ADHD

Drinking and Smoking in Pregnancy Period

Deadly alcohol and tobacco exposure are believed to perform a role in ADHD. Kids who are prenatally subjected to cigarette smoke are 2.4 times more probable to have ADHD than people who are not, evidence indicates. "Fetuses subjected to alcohol may produce fetal alcohol or fetal alcohol disorder, and the signs you see of ADHD are common with both," said Mark L. Wolraich, MD, director of the Developmental as well as Behavioral Pediatrics division at the Institution of Oklahoma medical sciences complex, Oklahoma town.

Exposure to Lead

Neurotoxic substance lead has been eliminated from several households and classrooms but there are still signs of it everywhere. A 2009 research showed that kids with ADHD appeared to have higher rates of blood-leads than other adolescents. "Lead may be toxic to the development of brain tissue could have maintained impact on the development of exposing kids to such substances at an early age," said Leavitt, who is practicing under Richard Oelberger 's supervision. "Still, such exposure is unlikely to account for brain differences advancement in the large majority of ADHD kids and teens."

Food Flavorings

After research, several European states have banned specific additives, which connected impulsivity in small kids to food only with blends of some and sodium preservative benzoic. The FDA said that when utilized "correctly," dietary supplements are safe, but most additives are not required to be evidently labeled on the packaging. Experts believe that a small percentage of kids will benefit from trying to avoid brightly colored foods that are processed and appear to have even more preservatives. "Seek advice with your kid's doctor before you put your kid on a specific diet," Leavitt says. Reducing the utilize of such preservatives may not contribute to excitable behavior; in ADHD, many factors play a key role.

Sugar Intake

Mother and father often blame the excitable behavior of a kid for sugar but it is time to stop it. "The overpowering numerous studies have failed to show behavioral changes in kids due to sugar intake," said Dr. Wolraich. An investigation published in the journal of such unusual kid development found that women who thought that sugar was given to their kids assessed the behavior of their kids as being more excitable than moms who were told that a sugar substitute was given to their kids — irrespective as to whether their kids actually ingested real sugar.

Video Games or TV

So, there's no evidence that ADHD is caused by much TV as well as video game time, even if the research has suggested that school-age and college and high school-age had much more attention difficulties than others who did not. The continuous exposure of television and video gaming will, in principle, make it easier for kids to pay focus. And yet experts stress that only screen time didn't comprehend ADHD. There's an affiliation between the (ADHD) and the number of more hour's young kids watch TV as well as play computer games, but much more study is needed to determine whether it's a causal connection or because kids with ADHD are gravitating more towards those actions," said by Dr. Wolraich.

Bad Kid Parenting

Symptoms of ADHD may be associated as disruptive or inappropriate conduct, and it's not unusual to seek to pin a kid's actions on the mother. But there is no significant evidence, as per the statewide counseling center at ADHD, too that authoritative parenting leads to ADHD.

"Although it's clear that authoritative parenting and social conditions can exacerbate ADHD habits, authoritative parenting is not the trigger of ADHD," said by Leavitt, that says family and friends who may have specific behavioral boundaries, using incentive and outcome behavioral strategies, and have a simple range of goals will help minimize symptoms of ADHD.

Injuries of Brain

"Head trauma that occurs from a heavy stroke to the head, either neurological disorder, an injury, or illness may trigger inattention issues and impaired control of physical function and tendencies," Leavitt notes. But due to the community mental wellbeing Institute, kids with some forms of brain damage can have signs close to ADHD. But since only a limited percentage of adolescents with ADHD also experienced brain trauma, this is not deemed a significant risk indicator.

Heredity

The research clearly shows that caregivers pass on the ADHD, not the parental method.

"ADHD possesses a very proud legacy," Smith affirms. "It is perhaps one of the greatest inherited psychological conditions." Indeed, a kid is 4 times more likely to seems to have had a close relative who also was given a diagnosis with ADHD, and the results of various twin studies signify that ADHD frequently occurs in families. Continuing work seeks to classify the genes that are responsible more for ADHD. The latest analysis mostly by researchers at the University of Cardiff in Wales reported that kids to ADHD are far more actually likely to have more lacking or overlapped DNA segments.

Notes:

Chapter 4:   ADHD Treatment

Treating ADHD With Medication

Treatment is aimed at changing or controlling behaviors that interfere with daily life, relationships, and professional ambitions. In most cases, medication will be used to improve concentration, irritability, and hyperactivity. Many children do much better in school when on medication.

It sounds counterproductive to give someone who is hyperactive and easily distracted a stimulant, but these medications have a very soothing effect on someone suffering from this disorder. Some of the most commonly prescribed stimulants include:

- Adderall

- Concerta

- Ritalin

- Daytrana

There are different forms of stimulant medications. For example, there are three forms of Ritalin: Ritalin, Ritalin SR, Ritalin LA. Doctors, or psychiatrists must consider the symptoms experienced by a patient to determine which stimulants will be the most effective without risking negative side effects.

In most cases side effects for stimulants are not severe. Many stimulants are known to curb appetite, so children must be watched closely to ensure they do not lose too much weight or stop eating. Some sufferers may have trouble sleeping on certain stimulants.

A Parent's Worst Nightmare

If the side effects of medication are typically so minor, why are so many parents scared to put their children on ADHD medication? The problem is there have been too many stories of children becoming lifeless robots without any sign of emotion or personality. This can become a problem when children are placed on the wrong medications or are given dosages that are too high.

Parents have to watch children on ADHD medication closely for any sign of personality change or tics. Tics are involuntary movement that looks like a spasm or jerk. It can occur in any body part. If parents can catch the development of tics or personality change, the dosage or medication can be adjusted to hopefully correct the side effect.

These potential side effects are a risk of taking medication for ADHD. Adults can watch themselves for negative side effects, but parents have the tough job of watching their children and deciding when a medication is working or when it may need adjusted or changed.

Behavior Management for Children

Behavior management is simply a form of psychotherapy. A therapist will work with a child to identify behavioral symptoms of ADHD that are making their life more difficult, or which may be interfering with their social or school life. They will then teach the child strategies to control and correct these behaviors when they notice them occurring.

While medication covers up the symptoms of ADHD, behavior management allows children to take control of those symptoms and overcome them. Most kids feel empowered when they go through this process, because there is something, they can do to correct the behaviors that stand in their way of making friends, being successful in school, and reaching other goals.

The Difficult Times

All children struggle through difficult times in their lives, but children with ADHD may have more trouble getting through major life changes. A therapist often becomes a safe outlet for emotions, so they do not build up and cause behavior problems in daily life. The behavioral symptoms of ADHD that interfere with daily life can easily become bigger problems when a child is going through a stressful time.

This is when working with a therapist to control behavior becomes very important. Children learn how to control their own behavior even when they are under intense stress or are dealing with other emotions.

Social Interactions

Many children with ADHD struggle socially. A therapist may work extensively on basic social skills, such as taking turns and accepting the differences in others. Some children need help reading the nonverbal cues that other children give when communicating, and some may need help understanding tones of voice as well. All children have to learn these things, but children with ADHD often need some extra help in interacting successfully with others.

Learning to Reward

Therapists will often encourage children to reward themselves in a healthy manner when they are able to control or overcome specific behavioral symptoms of ADHD. This helps repair self-confidence, which can be quite low in children suffering from ADHD.

These children are often punished in school and at home for behaviors that feel out of their control, so it helps to reward themselves as they see that they can control those behaviors. They have a higher sense of self control and while rewarding themselves, they feel better about themselves.

Help from Medication

Some children suffer more from hyperactivity, while others suffer more from the mental aspects of ADHD, such as lack of focus. Those with hyperactivity and other behavioral symptoms will respond best to psychotherapy. Those with more mental symptoms may need to rely more on medication to control those symptoms. For most children, a mix of behavioral management and mediation is the perfect solution.

Notes:

Chapter 5: ADHD at an Early Age

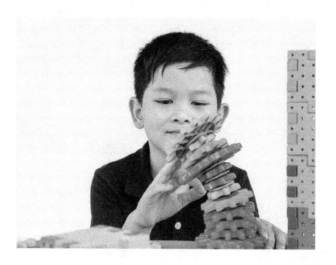

Children who are born with Attention Deficit Hyperactivity Disorder or ADHD have many different needs that tend to change with age and surroundings. These strategies and tips will help you understand your child better and help him lead a rewarding life.

Mornings are hectic for all parents as they are responsible for getting their children to school with tidy clothes, properly filled backpacks, and a decent breakfast. For such parents and children, the morning, and perhaps the rest of the day, can be quite chaotic. ADHD is a neurological disorder that makes the patient disorganized, impulsive, and easily bored or distracted.

Generally, ADHD is diagnosed when the child is in third grade, but in some cases, it can be diagnosed earlier. Parenting is already a difficult task for many, but parenting ADHD children can be quite a complex, challenging, and impulsive task. Parents who have ADHD children need to be on their toes all the time. Such parents have to be 'super-parents'. There are many tips, strategies, methods and information given in the book that can help you become a super-parent and raise a healthy, active, and smart child.

Let us first have a look at early age children and ADHD.

ADHD In Preschool

Do you think that your high-energy kid may have ADHD?

Many parents face this dilemma nearly every day. This is not because of the prevalence of the disorder, rather it is because almost all young kids i.e. preschoolers are almost always fidgety, impulsive, inattentive, and cranky. Many child psychiatrists and scientists who have studied preschoolers have concluded this. Instead of worrying about your kid and assuming the worst, it is recommended to talk to a medical professional.

Consult a pediatrician if you think that your child's behavior is impairing his ability to socialize, learn, and be safe. If anyone of the above three facets are jeopardized, you should consult a medical professional immediately, or else it could lead to other problems. Other signs of ADHD include extreme impulsiveness, excessive aggression, fidgetiness, etc. For instance, if your children can't wait for their turn, grab things that they are not allowed to touch, or perform activities that can harm them or others around them physically, it is necessary to consult a doctor.

If your preschooler has ADHD, your first focus needs to be improving your parenting skills. For instance, going to PCIT or Parent-Child Interaction Therapy can help you understand how to your child's behavior. It is generally a two to three-month-long therapy period in which a therapist observes you while you and your children play together. This observation is done with the help of a one-way mirror and you receive instructions through an earpiece. This method can work wonders for your relationship with your child and can make both your child and you feel comfortable, happy and better about each other.

Talk to a child psychologist (or the therapist available at the school) and check whether you should use this therapy or any other behavioral therapy to break barriers with your child.

Tips

Feedback

Always offer positive feedback whenever your child follows the rules and obeys orders.

Bad Behavior

Do not give in to bad behavior ever. Even if your child starts to act up in public, do not give in to his demands out of sheer embarrassment. Instead, just leave the place without him and he will follow you.

Stimulation

Reduce his TV time, computer game time etc. Just an hour is sufficient at that age; otherwise it might lead to sensory overload.

Social Burnout

Do not let his socialization skills burnout. Reduce his play date time, especially whenever you feel he is getting along with his playdate. End the playdate, whenever he wants more time, which you can use as a bargaining chip for positive behavior.

Energy

Add a few high-energy activities in his daily schedule. This way he will burn extra energy off in a safe and controlled environment. It is recommended to schedule such activities during the daytime and not just a couple of hours before bedtime.

Notes:

Chapter 6: The Do's and Don'ts of Parenting A Child With ADHD

Almost every parent of an ADHD child knows that having the condition may explain bad behavior, but doesn't provide an excuse to get away with it without any consequences.

There are special challenges for treating the ADHD child in a way that can help them to understand the consequences of their actions. The main thing is to deal with the negative behavior at the time it occurs so that it does not escalate.

Some reportedly successful methods include:

Direct Contact

Direct Contact doesn't mean physical punishment. It refers to gently setting your hands on each side of your child's face, looking him or her in the eye, and saying his name until you have full attention.

The child soon realizes he has no choice but to focus, listen, and pay attention to what you are saying. Obviously, this method won't work if your child is in the middle of a full-blown tantrum, but in most cases, by being vigilant, you will be able to stop that from happening.

Don't Over-Explain

Many modern mothers have a misguided, if admirable habit of trying to explain decisions or prohibitions to their children, even to their ADHD children. This is liable to drive your ADHD child into a screaming fit, particularly if already frustrated and upset. Keep it simple and consistent. Focus on what needs to be done, right "now". In this way, you will not waste your breath and you can nip the negative behavior in the bud as quickly as 1-2-3.

If you are consistent with your rules and regulations, then there is never any need to explain.

Reward Positive Behavior

Expect your child to behave as a matter of course, no matter what medical condition they might or might not have. Don't ever excuse them on the grounds of their health. Let your child know what you expect, and reward them when they do it.

A simple word of praise will do it: "Great listening, Eileen!" Make sure the praise is sincere, however, and not repeated by rote, or it will quickly become meaningless.

By rewarding good behavior instead of punishing bad behavior, your child will be more eager to please. Conversely, a child who feels they can never do anything right will just give up and get worse if you are too exacting in your standards.

Your goal is to get your child to progress as much as possible without leaving you and them frustrated, so reward them for what they can do and sandwich chores or tasks that your child finds difficult between ones they enjoy.

Sandwich Chores and Tasks

Since your child's attention span will be limited, be sure that their work offers variety in a short amount of time and then move on to the next task.

Also try to sandwich tasks they don't like or are not that good at with ones that they do. If they are bad at math, do not start or finish their homework session with that subject, as it can quickly lead them to a frustrated impasse on the one hand, or to give up on the other. Get them to start out with their favorite subject, and then do a small number of math problems. Do another couple of problems, and then swap tasks again. In this way, it helps the time to pass and they won't feel so restless or trapped at the prospect of a long homework session on a subject they dislike.

Keep to Your Own Rules

It's amazing the number of parents who set their child a bad example, and then are frustrated and angry when their ADHD child does the same thing. One has to be extra careful in this area, because ADHD children don't catch all the nuances that might make a decision acceptable for an adult, but not for a child.

In addition, it is essential that you be consistent. If there is to be no television after nine o'clock on a school night, that means all the children, all the time, not some of the children, some of the time. This can be difficult if you have older children, so allow their privileges to be age-appropriate, but remember that they are just that, privileges, not rights.

Children learn a great deal by example. ADHD children will make observations and often jump to incorrect conclusions, so be consistent and do not have any disputes in front of them regarding care or privileges. Everyone in the family should support the family schedule, routine, and rules of the household.

Use Time-Outs

This involves isolating the child in a room or corner without distracting material to punish them. Keep it very short when first introducing them to the concept.

Make the number of minutes equate with the child's age and do not enter into any discussion or argument. Warn them, and if the bad behavior persists, tell them they have to sit on the naughty chair or in the corner for X minutes until they calm down.

When the time is up, explain to them briefly why they were there. In most cases they will be happy to say they are sorry and join in again. Sending a child to their room with no follow up is the worst thing you can do to try to discipline a child. No matter how frustrated or angry you are, try to keep your emotions out of your disciplinary strategies and be consistent and firm.

Make Consequences Immediate

Children are very immediate creatures. They have usually forgotten the bad behavior they did at the time the punishment rolls around.

ADHD children are even more inclined this way. Therefore, if you delay punishment for misbehavior until later, you're inviting

148

drama, conflict, emotion, and an unpleasant and exhausting experience for all involved. They will feel the punishment is coming out of the blue and is unfair.

If there is to be a time out or a punishment such as the removal of a privilege, make it immediate. For example, if they are grounded from television, turn off the television immediately. State how long the punishment will last. Make it reasonable so that they can remember and not just shrug it off as "never" getting the television back. Say, "You kicked your brother twice, even after I told you that is not the way we behave in this home. You are not allowed to watch television for the rest of the evening."

Naturally, the other children might also end up deprived, so you might need to give them a time out in another room and give them something useful to do.

Put the Responsibility Back on Your Own Child

For older children, if your child has "messed up", immediately tell them what the main issue is, and ask them: "What are you going to do to fix this?"

For example, if they were fidgeting around in the house and broke a vase that you treasured, ask them what they are going to do to fix it. They could try to glue it back together, though that can be a bit unsafe and not always practical.

They might also offer to do extra chores to help pay for a new one. (Children should always get pocket money in proportion to their chores, not a guaranteed allowance. In this way, they will be less likely to take for granted what you give them.)

Then wait for their response to the question, and help them come up with a plan. This is probably the only occasion when it is better to ask a question about disruptive behavior. Usually, questions just distract and lead to drama.

Putting the responsibility appropriately back on them when it is age-appropriate seems to be the best way to help ADHD children understand that there are consequences to their negative behavior towards others, and that they have to take responsibility for their own actions.

Remember, ADHD children are pretty much "black and white" in their thinking. Since they lack the ability to perceive nuances in situations, and most young people can see only good and bad, keep it simple. Make clear rules, and make sure you stick to them yourself. Apply them consistently to all the children in your family, and make sure that any caregivers helping you do the same.

What Doesn't Work with Children Who Have ADHD

There is a growing body of evidence about what will work best if you wish to communicate effectively with a child who has ADHD, and about what will not work and should be avoided.

It may be unfashionable to say this, but modern parents seem to think that it is a good idea to be their child's buddy or best friend. Sorry, but your role is to be the parent.

Many people shy away from being too dictatorial or black and white with their children, but there is nothing wrong with being clear about your expectations with respect to behavior, and expecting your children to meet your expectations.

It is your job to socialize your child as a responsible parent so that they will get along well with others and within a variety of situations in life. Your child will not love you any less for expecting them to be the best they can be. The point is rewarding their efforts, and the fact that they try, even if they do not succeed.

With a child with ADHD, you need to be very clear about what you expect and want at all times, even if it goes against your notion of more liberal parenting. Here are several things that will not work and should be avoided once you are sure that your child has ADHD:

- Argument and Reasoning

- Asking Questions When Giving Commands

- Constant Criticism and Negativity towards Your Child

- Being Too Lenient

- Basing Your Expectations on Your Moods

- Punishing Your Child in a Way that They Can't Understand

- Not Being Consistent from Day to Day and from Caregiver to Caregiver

Notes:

Chapter 7: Disciplining Kids With ADHD

Keep Calm and Carry On was the catchphrase used by the British government at the beginning of WWII to spur on its citizens. It can also be used as the motto for the parents of children who have ADHD. Parents of ADHD kids walk a fine line between being patient and being a disciplinarian, between allowing your child to develop as far as he/she can and protecting them from the disappointments that you know they will have to face. They all want to spare their children hurt but they also want them to learn to be strong. It is a very challenging job.

Extensive knowledge of the disorder and how it affects your child's functioning can help, when the time comes to discipline your child, because you will be able to discern the difference between conscious bad behavior and behavior that is a result of ADHD. The more you know, the more you can work with your child to reach a happy medium. He or she must always know that they are loved no matter what they do or how they behave.

Discipline techniques used for other children might not work for children with ADHD, but there must be boundaries and codes of conduct established. The kid with ADHD needs a firm but loving hand when being corrected. You must fight to control your anger even when the child is displaying behavior that is clearly unacceptable, or is refusing to follow instructions. Removing privileges such as time playing computer games or looking at television is one way of dispensing discipline. Time outs are also a favorite for parents of children with ADHD. They should be put into effect as soon as the infringement is committed and should not last too long because the child won't be able to complete it, and the effect will be lost. You also have to be careful not to transfer your frustration at your ADHD child to your other children as they could end up being scolded a lot more severely than they deserved to be simply because you needed an outlet for your anger.

A sense of humor is very valuable in a home with a child with ADHD. You should learn to laugh instead of being embarrassed every time your child does things that might be socially unacceptable in a public place. It won't be easy but try to remember that in time the embarrassment will pass, and all that will be left would be a fun story to relate to your friends and relatives. Sometimes it is okay just to ignore the bad behavior once it is not causing anyone, including the child himself, any harm. This is not suggested as an ongoing way of dealing with the issue of tantrums and other forms of misbehavior, but sometimes it is the right thing to do. Children with ADHD need constant attention and to get it they would be willing to behavior badly because negative attention is still attention. If your child is complaining and arguing for no reason just ignore him until it stops. If the complaining accelerates, let the child know that you would not be responding until he clams down. Like everything else, this will be successful some of the time but won't work in every instance. You will have to gauge when it is the right time to use it.

Your child is going to make many mistakes. Learn to compromise by letting the small one's pass. Pick your battles carefully and deal with issues individually. Don't try to solve every problem at once because that is setting yourself up for disappointment. Through all the challenges, never stop believing in your child and his ability to overcome. Make this clear to the child as well; he should know at all times that you believe in him. Stay positive. Encourage your child to vocalize his feelings. If he is able to tell you when he is feeling sad or angry, you might be able to help him in addressing the problem before it leads to an episode of bad behavior. Because children with ADHD are often disorganized and impulsive, they need a structured existence even more than others. Make the rules very clear to the child so he knows exactly what is expected of him. Break down instructions into simple steps and speak in the clearest and plainest of ways. Make him repeat what you said back to you so you know that he has heard it. Many parents have found it helpful to engage in role playing with their child in order to make the link for him between his behavior and the reaction of his parent to it. Children with ADHD can often make that connection and establishing it can help in minimizing behavior that is unacceptable.

These rules may need explaining a bit more often than with other children, so you have to be patient but persistent and keep repeating the limits until they get it. Make the child understand that if the rules aren't followed there will be consequences such as no television or spending time in his room, and if need be those consequences will be implemented.

Find ways within yourself to also remain calm. Confrontations with your child can be an exercise in patience and tolerance for you and the child. Ensure that the consequences of bad behavior do not cause the child undue distress but are in proportion to the offense. Don't get carried away with the withdrawal of privileges to the point where you are taking away things that are major events in the child's life. Don't say for instance that you are going to cancel his birthday party.

Before you can begin disciplining a child with ADHD, you have to know what behaviors the child can control and which he cannot. Offer rewards to the child for compliance with rules and for following instructions. Discipline for an ADHD child, even more so than an ordinary child, should never involve spanking, beating or any form of violence. Make sure they understand what they did that was unacceptable, and if possible, have them redress the wrong, for example, apologizing to another child or cleaning up a mess they made.

Don't try to suppress all the child's efforts at independence. A little defiance might be a positive sign that your child is trying to deal with the world on his own terms. You don't want to take away all his spirit because he is going to need it to cope with the obstacles that he will face growing up.

One of the first things a parent has to learn to do is to censor him or herself. When you are tempted to coddle your child and be his buffer against the world, remember that that child also has to grow and learn to deal with the world on his own. The disorder is not going to go away, it is going to stay with him into adulthood, but at some point, in his life you will no longer be there and he will have to be able to fend for himself and get along in the world.

It is important to put structure into the lives of children with ADHD by setting down rules and establishing limits of acceptable behavior. Try not to be too rigid or to set deadlines and standards that cause rebellion and confrontation. Still give your child a feeling of independence albeit within boundaries.

Although parents should expect some disobedience as with any child, there must be consequences when the child does not follow the rules. Don't assume that his behavior is because of the disorder and cannot be controlled. Although most of the time this will be the case, children with ADHD, like other children, will push as far as they can until their parents stop them. Sometimes unacceptable behavior is deliberate. Stick to your guns. It will probably take longer to get your child with ADHD to comply with your structure than the average child, but you must not give up on them or on the schedule that you have set. Even playtime can be used as a learning tool if used correctly. Use puzzles and other brain stimulating toys when you play with your child. This way he can be learning while enjoying play and spending time with a parent all at once.

Even though you have to instill discipline in your child's life, try to minimize negative feedback and comments. Chances are the child gets enough negativity in his daily life already. Try to teach the way to do things using as much positive and as little negative reinforcement as possible. Any improvement in behavior must be loudly applauded. If the only time that the child gets any attention is when he does something wrong and the rest of the time he is ignored, he will continue to do the wrong thing. Let him know that good behavior can bring him lots of attention too and even better if it is positive attention. When correcting your child, be sure to explain in the plainest terms exactly what he has done that is wrong and why it is wrong. Of course, this is easier said than done.

After telling your kid numerous times not to leave his skateboard on the stairs but to put it away in the closet under the stairs, if you almost trip over it as you come down the stairs on your way to work, it is very easy to lose your temper and to begin shouting. Try however to think ahead to what the outcome of that might be. You'll shout and the child will respond by either being crushed or being defiant and shouting back. If he's defiant, that will increase your anger, there'll be more shouting from both sides and general bad behavior will ensue most likely ending with a timeout for the child.

You will feel guilty because you lost your temper and shouted and because you can't seem to get him to carry out what is a very simple instruction. Meanwhile, the skateboard will still be on the stairs waiting to trip someone.

So instead of going through all that, rein in your anger, sit your little one down and explain to him why leaving it there is dangerous, and why there must be consequences to his failure to remember to put it away. Make sure that he understands the issue; keep explaining until he gets it.

Notes:

Chapter 8: Food to Eat to Help Them Grow Healthy

Recent studies by Yunus (2019) from the renowned Exceptional Parent have asserted how there is a possible link between ADHD and high sugar, salt, and fat intake when kids receive diets with only minimal whole grains, fruits and vegetables intakes (p. 24). Many findings specifically herald the benefits of a whole food plant-based (WFPB) diet with minimal or no processing for protection against ADHD, cancers, heart disease, osteoporosis, and other chronic conditions (Yunus, 2019, p. 24) as well.

Are you ready for some yummy suggestions? Let us find those aprons, ok?

Snack Attacks: Make snack attacks healthy with fresh fruits and veggies. Make healthy smoothies together and add some chia and flax seeds to balance moods. Masterchef Junior, anyone?

Mr. and Ms. Clean: This advice does not mean operating a pristine household free of dust bunnies and flawlessness, but it is about eating as clean as possible to avoid unnecessary additives and food colorings. Of course, kids are attracted to the colorful, marshmallow, vibrant products that are often so full of crap. Yunus (2019) also divulges how we have a clear responsibility as parents and the ones who typically purchase the food products to ensure that nutrition is clean for children, tweens, and teens with ADHD since "This is a controversial subject and, because we often have an emotional attachment to food, we are reluctant to look at this as an adjunct treatment" (p. 25).

Diggity D: There is "No Diggity" about it that Vitamin D is the superior sunlight vitamin that most kids, tweens, and teens often lack from excessive indoor gadget time, nutritional voids, etc. As a result, Laliberte's (2010) "Problem Solved: Winter Blues" from Prevention insists that we must all ensure that our family members are digging it with vitamin D proactively since it is closely linked to keeping our serotonin levels elevated and balanced (p. 48). This connection is something that is super important in kids, tweens, and teens with ADHD for critical brain balance and overall wellness.

Are you excited to dig it with D? Take a family hike, jog, stroll, or skate around the block. Find a local park and dive into the D!

Straight from the Hive: Try warm milk with Manuka honey for a natural relaxer before bedtime with your kiddos. My girls really love it on bananas with peanut butter and chia seeds, too. You can also add it to evening herbal teas to evoke some sweet dreams and deeper sleep.

As a slight disclaimer, because of honey's sugary contents, be sure to just use a small amount, roughly the size of a poker chip. Just do not try to karaoke Lady Gaga's "Poker Face" song, or you might lose face with older kids! BEE holistic, BEE well, and BEE wonderful when you try honey with your honey!

Sugar High: As adults, we really need to embrace the "You are what you eat" mindset with all kids, but especially those who have ADHD. In turn, closely monitor sugar intake with their candies, sodas, caffeinated beverages, and all those ooey gooey treats and desserts. Carefully monitor the amount of fast foods that you are serving to your families, not matter how tempting or timesaving it may seem. Studies encourage us to eat "clean" as clean as possible as opposed to relying on the fatty, greasy, overprocessed foods. Clean eating will naturally "eliminate unnecessary food additives such as artificial colors, flavors, sweeteners, and preservatives that do not add nutritional value and may contribute to ADHD symptoms. Limit sugar intake to 10% of total calories daily (roughly 6 teaspoons for children aged 2 to 19 years)" (Rucklidge, Taylor, & Johnstone, 2018, p. 16).

Putting a freeze on fast food addictions can be so instrumental. La Valle's (1998) pioneering article from Drug Store News also indicates how high sugar intakes can cause low blood sugar and chromium depletion. The fast food frenzy is really taking a toll on our kids as "The average American now consumes an average of 152.5 pounds of sugar in a year. That large soft drink at the drive-through window contains roughly 22 to 27 teaspoonfuls of sugar. It is reported that increased sugar intake actually increases urinary chromium excretion. Over time, this could have an impact on behavior" (CP13).

MOOve Over: Dairy overload can often cause major digestive issues. When kids are literally plugged up, they can act out even more. To counter these tummy troubles, consider some new dairy alternatives like almond, soy, coconut, cashew, and oat milk. I also suggest adding probiotics to your kiddos' diets with more kefir, Greek yogurt, and other mood foods. In my daughters' cases, they have been extremely helpful to tame tummies and boost moods. Let us MOOve over mindfully!

Veg Heads: You can opt for a Meatless Monday approach for more mindful family eating. Try to replace traditional noodles with veggies such as asparagus, zucchini, carrots, etc. Indulge in Brussel sprouts, cauliflower pizza crust, corns, asparagus, etc. Be a vicious veg head and also add more veggies to morning egg dishes, especially omelets.

Make the Jolly Green Giant proud and be a veg head of household more often to facilitate holistic health and happiness in all kids, but especially ones with ADHD! My oldest daughter adores making and eating kale chips with me. She has also recently been trying the freeze-dried snap peas, too. We never know what they will like until we experiment, right? Go beyond broccoli and green beans on your next grocery run!

In essence, it is also highly advantageous to ensure that your kids are getting enough B vitamins in their diets: B1 is linked closely to many key functions like immunity, heart support, and mental processing; B2 offers energy, hair, skin, and eye health; B 3 stabilizes our memories, moods, and hearts; B5 can keep cholesterol levels in check; B6 is a sleep reliever. Are you ready for some "Sweet Dreams" by Queen Bey?

Finally, buzz with B-12 for increased mood and energy management. My young kids love the "classic ants on a log" snack with peanut butter, cashew butter, sunflower seed butter, or almond butter slathered onto celery with raisins, dried cherries, or cranberries. Have fun in the kitchen and make Rachael Ray proud in a healthy and mindful way today!

Beanie: While I am not talking about the cool, fashionable hats, try to eat more mindfully against ADHD with beans and legumes. Make black beans burritos, hummus with chick-peas, serve up some edamame, and add lentils or sunflower seeds to beam up your families' diets!

Magnesium Magnets: Strive to add more magnesium into your family's overall dietary routines, especially in cases of ADHD. Studies describe how the average American is often highly deficient in magnesium "by about 70 mg daily. Magnesium is the calming mineral, since it is the principal mineral used to control the parasympathetic nervous system. There is also the potential for calcium deficiency. Many children complain of aching legs and will see positive results with the initiation of a well formulated multiple mineral supplement" (La Valle, 1998, CP13.). Get your magnesium magnets via food or supplements today!

In fact, salmon nuggets and fish sticks are always major hits with my girls! They also enjoy coconut shrimp with fun and tasty dipping sauces. How can you get your Nemo and Dory on and blast more fish in your weekly menus?

See for Yourself: Fruits like pineapples, grapefruits, tomatoes, berries, mangoes, oranges, and kiwis, are a definite self-care saver for the blasts of vitamin C. I also recently discovered passion fruit, a rich source of beta-carotene and vitamin C, as recommended by the recent article aptly called "Mood Food" (2019) from Daily Mail.

My girls love to toss some seeds onto their morning yogurt parfaits. Try some today and see for yourself if your kids will likely say "Yay!"

Zing with Zinc: Assist your kids with ADHD in the culinary department to better zing against mood swings, common colds, flus, and other physical problems. Simply add more fruits and vegetables rich in zinc to their diets daily.

Honor the great pumpkin! Don't wait for Halloween and toss some pumpkin seeds to kids' sandwiches, baked goods, cereals, oatmeal, yogurts, pastas, salads, etc. Experts praise them for reducing feelings of anxiety (Mood Food, 2018), something that kids, tweens, and teens with ADHD know all too well, right? Let's zing and sing with zinc!

Grain Brains: Apply more whole grains to your family's meals regularly. Go for wheat breads, overnight oats, brown rice and pastas, quinoa, barely, granola, etc. Gravitate toward making some grain brain nutritional gains!

Happy and Hydrated: I know you have probably heard this one a zillion times, but it is vital to reiterate the value of ensuring that kids get enough water daily. If your kids will not drink water plain, have fun adding cucumber slices, lime, lemon, berries, mint, or other fun and tasty additions. Let us hoot for hydration happily and holistically!

Notes:

Chapter 9:   Great Activities and Playground Safety

School is a great way to keep ADHD kids busy, but about summer breaks and winter? During summer, there is no homework to keep kids occupied, and the hot afternoons can stretch on forever. It is too cold for kids to play outdoors in the winter, which led to days of whining, complaining, and boredom. There are many ways to keep kids occupied at home. These tried-and-tested activities can stimulate the active imaginations of ADHD children and keep them out of trouble when school's out

Bird watching

If you live in an area with lots of greens and wildlife, bird-watching is a great way to keep kids occupied. Look at the pictures of birds in your area and challenge your kid to spot these birds and write down the species they've seen. You can also do bird-related activities like creating a simple bird feeder. Get a 2-liter plastic bottle and cut out a hole in the center where birds can go in and out. Create two smaller holes below the large hole and stick a branch through the center – this will be a place where birds can sit. At the bottle's neck create two small holes to thread nylon strings through. Fill the bottle with bird seed and hang it by the string onto a tree branch.

Grow a garden

Spring and summer is a great time to grow a garden. Even those living in the city can make a small garden on a balcony or fire escape. A garden is not only a great way to get your child outdoors;

it will teach him or her how to be responsible. Let your child take care of the garden every day and to write down the changes that happen to the plants. He or she can write down every time the plant grows a new blossom or bears fruit.

Treasure hunting

The treasure hunt game is a fun activity you can do indoors, especially if you had two children or more. Using simple "treasures" from a dollar store, ask your kids to hide these objects all over the house. Have each child draw a treasure map that leads to each item. Once they're done making their maps, have your kids exchange maps and locate the items they hid.

Pen pals

If you have friends or relatives who live in different parts of the country or abroad see if they have children who are your children's ages. If they do, set up a pen pal network among children so each can learn about the how the other lives and the things they do.

Dress-up box

Using un-wanted clothes or chose, create a dress-up box that your kids can use for Halloween, school plays, and games that require costumes. You can also scour yard sales and thrift stores for fun items to add to dress-up box.

Coping Skills and Physical Activity

Coping skills will vary from child to child, as with everything else. Some skills can be learned from therapists, while other skills come from physical activity, a favorite past-time such as engaging in creative play, video games, and schedules. Your ADHD child is in need of many different coping skills, so I hope to give you some valuable tools for your parental "toolbox" to pass along to your child.

Coping skills from therapists are often gained through play therapy, but if this isn't an option for your family, my suggestion would be to find something your child enjoys, then encourage the child to use this option when they feel they are losing control. If playing with clay keeps your child's attention put a plastic tablecloth on the kitchen table and let him/her go wild. You can even give them a task, such as making a flower, dinosaur, gingerbread man, etc. to keep things interesting. When the project is finished, let it dry out, then place it somewhere prominent in the home or in your child's room to help build self-esteem.

Physical activity is always a plus for the ADHD child. When you notice your child is becoming hyperactive, have them go outside (weather permitting!) and run around the house two or three times and repeat as necessary, LOL! Seriously, though, ANY type of physical activity such as shooting baskets, running, jumping jacks, playing volleyball, bike riding, etc. will be helpful in bringing your child's hyperactivity under control.

If your child enjoys video games, make sure you are purchasing age-appropriate games, as well as games that challenge the child's mind. Games containing puzzles to be unlocked before moving to the next level help teach patience build self-confidence. Educational games that can teach critical thinking or math skills, or games that encourage your child to use their imagination are all beneficial in their own right. Something to keep in mind here is to NOT allow electronics to become a babysitter for your ADHD child. Limit game time for after finishing homework/chores, on the weekends for short periods, long car rides, or as an alternative to watching mindless television.

Playground Safety

Parks and playgrounds provide fun, fresh air, and lots of exercise. But some playgrounds can also pose some hazards if parents are not careful and aware of playground's safety measure. Every year nearly 300,000 children get into accidents on the playground due to improper surfaces, faulty equipment, and careless behavior.

As you are probably aware, children with ADHD tend to be more accident-prone than the rest because of their impulsive behavior and hyperactive tendencies. That's why it's important for you to keep your child safe on the playground. Here are a few things you can do.

Supervise your child

Make sure your child stays safe by supervising your child or making sure an adult is around to keep an eye on the kids. Adult supervision prevents injuries by making sure kids use playground equipment properly and don't do unsafe activities near other children. This is important because young children have difficulty in gauging distances; older children, on the other hand, like to test their limits playground equipment. Even if an adult cannot prevent injuries, at least he or she can administer first aid immediately or take the child to the emergency room.

Dress your child in play clothes

Make sure your child doesn't wear long necklaces or hoodies and pants with drawstrings. They can lead to injuries by catching onto equipment, or can accidentally strangle a child.

Evaluate the fall surfaces

Approximately 70% of playground injuries are due to falls. One-way to prevent them is make sure the fall surfaces of playground equipment are properly cushioned. Make sure that the surfaces around swings, seesaws, and sliders are softened using wood chips, sand mulch, pea gravel, or rubber. Concrete surfaces are unsafe, and so are grass or soil-packed surfaces; regular wear and tear can reduce their cushioning capacities.

Teach your child about playground safety

Safe equipment and adult presence are important but they're not enough to prevent injuries. The other half of the equation is for your child to know how to stay safe on the playground. Some basic playground safety rules you can teach are:

- Use the equipment properly – don't stand on swings, slide feet first, one child per seat on the seesaw, etc.
- Do not push other kids while on the slides, swings, seesaws, or jungle gyms.
- Before jumping down, make sure no children are in the way. Always land on both feet with knees bent slightly.
- Do not use playground equipment after rain; the moisture will make the surface slippery.

Notes:

Chapter 10:   Practical and Loving Parenting

Parenting a child with ADHD requires flexibility, invention, and a great deal of patience, not only with your child but also with yourself. While you will go on to help your child using the strategies this discusses, it is important to realize that ADHD requires long-term management. Yes, the symptoms will improve, but the disorder will not just go away overnight. In some cases, it can be a lifelong condition.

Parenting Principles

As you help your child develop strategies to work with ADHD, there are several principles to keep in mind. These principles will help you guide your child in a realistic and caring way, with an understanding that there is no cure-all for ADHD. The guidance you provide can help your child work at their own pace toward understanding the condition and working with it.

Practice patience:

All parents need patience, and this quality is particularly important for parents of children with ADHD. While it is natural for parents to want to "solve" their children's problems and "cure" their ADHD, the reality for most children is that they need time to develop. Studies conducted by the NIMH and others have shown that children with ADHD will develop in similar ways as that of their peers, except in brain development, where they lag behind about three years. These studies suggest that parents can be assured that their children will eventually develop the necessary organizational, planning, and judgment skills exercised by children without ADHD. But, the slower trajectory toward maturation means extra patience and an eye on long-term development, rather than quick fixes, may be necessary.

Keep an eye on the long term:

This is related to patience. Parents should understand that even though they are taking steps to help their child, they might not see immediate results. Change and maturation require time, and children may develop more slowly in some areas than in others. They may experience occasional setbacks, but these bumps in their development do not mean that they won't eventually have all of the tools they require for a rich and productive life.

Ask others for help:

While it is natural for parents to want to help their children on their own, it really does "take a village" to raise all kids, particularly those with learning differences. In other words, reach out to a community of people who have children with ADHD, whether online or in your area, for advice and support. It is a positive reflection of your parenting style to enlist the help of adults your child interacts with, including not only teachers but also perhaps coaches, tutors, doctors, therapists, and religious leaders. Enlisting the help of others may be particularly important as your child enters adolescence, a period when children are often less receptive to what their parents have to say.

Externalize rewards:

As ADHD expert Russell Barkley, PhD, noted in Taking Charge of ADHD, children with ADHD may not internalize motivation as other children do over time, and they may need external motivations and supports to change their behavior. This does not mean that parents need to bribe children, but it does mean that parents need to consider what children with ADHD value, such as playing video games or sports, and use these interests as rewards for children's completion of more mundane activities. While many parents want children to carry out tasks just because it is the right thing to do, children with ADHD may need to be externally motivated until they can develop a more intrinsic sense of what they need to do over time.

Recognize positive behaviors:

Children with ADHD often require constant feedback. Be sure to recognize what your child is doing well, even if it's just part of a larger task or something trivial. For example, while most school-age children can get dressed and eat breakfast independently, many children with ADHD need to be praised for each step of the process they complete on their own—for instance, putting on their socks or tying their shoes without help, or sitting at the table for ten minutes without fidgeting. Though many parents may feel that children should not be praised for tasks that are expected of them at a certain age, children with ADHD need this praise to motivate them to keep completing these tasks on their own. It may feel strange to praise children who are still developing skill sets that their peers have already incorporated—or which parents think are easy—but it is necessary to keep children with ADHD moving toward independence. Big leaps can happen in very unexpected time frames, and little changes happen all the time; be unconditionally supportive of your child, and notice when they succeed regardless of how trivial the accomplishment may seem to you.

Break down tasks and directions into smaller parts:

Children with ADHD often need longer tasks and directions broken down into smaller, easier to manage pieces. Parents, teachers, and other caregivers should avoid assuming that a child with ADHD will understand how to break down longer tasks on their own. For example, in the morning, your child may need a list of each task they need to complete. An example might look like this: (1.) Take your clothes out of your drawer. (2.) Put on your clothes starting with your socks, etc. School assignments need to be broken down similarly. Also, specific times for completion need to be assigned, as many children with ADHD do not have an intrinsic sense of how to plan or complete tasks within a certain time frame.

Communicate with teachers and other professionals:

Children with ADHD have a legal right to special accommodations at school, including an Individualized Education Program (IEP), to help them succeed. However, many parents attempt to conceal an ADHD diagnosis, fearing that their child will be stigmatized. If they are not aware of the diagnosis, teachers and others in teaching and caregiving roles may assume a child is being willfully defiant or disruptive. If you communicate honestly about what your child is facing, this information will help teachers work with your child. Parents should not ask teachers to excuse their children from assignments. Instead, they should strategize with teachers about how to help their child complete the schoolwork.

Avoid comparing children to others, including siblings:

Children with ADHD already have an acute sense of not measuring up, and these types of comparisons, when shared with children, do not tend to motivate them. Comparisons for the purpose of trying to show your child with ADHD how they should behave can frustrate them further and lead to less self-confidence in working toward developing the skills they need.

Keep in mind the particular challenges of girls with ADHD:

While all children with ADHD may find that their symptoms interfere with positive social interactions, girls with ADHD may run afoul of cultural stereotypes about the ways they should behave. For example, they may be considered odd, socially distractible, too brusque, bossy, or other qualities that society— including many children, parents, and teachers—are not taught to celebrate in girls.

Take advantage of ADHD's benefits and energy:

While there is no doubt that ADHD presents challenges, it also can confer a great sense of creativity, high energy, and often considerable charm. The old adage, "feed the hungry bee," is a good mantra for parents. Find what your child likes to do, and encourage them to do it. For example, let's say your child loves working with tools or taking things apart. Buy them a building set, perhaps, and see if your child might want to help you fix things around the house. In other words, find the activities and tasks they enjoy (or at least tolerate), and give them an out if there's a task they truly dislike. Who knows, given the choice, your child might discover a knack for folding laundry or thrive at the responsibility of ironing shirts!

Recognize and channel kids' interests:

Many children with ADHD have specialized areas of interest they can develop. For example, they may have difficulty completing their homework, but they might be motivated by sports, drama, or robotics. You can help your child develop skills in an area of high interest, and your child will be more motivated to develop independence and discipline in that area. For example, if your child enjoys singing, they might set a goal of performing at a school concert, and you can help them develop a practice regimen. This experience can help your child understand the importance of hard work and breaking down preparation over time into small, achievable steps. Your child might then be more willing to internalize these lessons when completing traditional homework.

Take personal time to recuperate:

Parents of children with ADHD may simply feel exhausted, disappointed, and even isolated at times. They need to remember to take good care of themselves, too. If possible, find time for yourself to reflect and just relax. You might also enjoy joining groups for parents of children with ADHD so you can share experiences and strategies with others who are going through similar experiences. Connecting with other parents who understand what you are going through can also help reduce any sense of isolation you might be feeling.

Notes:

Chapter 11:   Ignore Mild Misbehavior

Children with ADHD, unlike most kids, exhibit attention-seeking behavior. They want to be noticed. They want to be attended to. It doesn't matter to them if good or bad behavior gets the job done. However, when we give them attention when they do something wrong and not when they do something right, they start to assume that negative behavior is the way to go. They begin to depict more bad behavior which can make the mums and dads go mad.

Thus, this next parenting skill is more of an art where you deliberately ignore misbehavior in the hopes that they will give it up on their own.

Choosing to ignore certain behaviors doesn't mean you pay no attention to their distress or anger. If they genuinely seem in pain or emotionally-troubled, you need to be there for them. Ignoring mild misbehavior means that you ignore the way they are behaving, not how they are feeling. Attention, in itself, is a big positive reinforcement, even if it comes out of negative action. But when you choose to not give it to them purposely, they look for other ways to get it. Thus, it is important that good behavior gets attention every time it is noticeable to encourage it.

Ignoring mild misbehavior also discourages it from being repeated and prevents power struggles. Ever had a moment where your child dropped to the floor in a busy grocery store because they wanted something? Well, it is their way of getting attention. But yelling and shouting only makes it worse, doesn't it? It is because when we do that, we unknowingly give them the attention they seek. To save ourselves from further embarrassment, we let them have what they want, which in a way, reinforces that behavior. When you choose to ignore the temper tantrum and pretend that it isn't effective, they try other means to get to you. This is a silent yet strategic way of letting them know that being obnoxious won't get them the desired results.

Why Do You Need to Keep Your Cool?

Another thing that happens frequently with many parents raising a child with ADHD is that they lose their patience after some time. They resort to yelling, shouting, and setting harsh punishments in hope that it will prevent misbehavior. Sadly, it doesn't work that way. Remaining calm and keeping your cool, on the other hand, does!

It is researchers at Ohio State University who believe so. The study offered biological evidence that positive parenting - parenting without punishments or using care and compassion to deal with misbehavior – may help children with ADHD master their behaviors and emotions (Bell et al., 2017). The study included both children with developmental disorders and their parents. Theodore Beauchaine, the leading author of the study was surprised to report that the psychological impact of praises and compliments instead of shouting and criticizing were almost instant.

The responses of the participants were monitored and evaluated during a special intervention program. The intervention program offered small group sessions for children and parents. The parents learned how to respond to their children's behaviors and the children were taught some strategies for anger management, emotion regulation, and emotionally aware and appropriate social behaviors. The researchers assigned renowned therapists to work with ninety-nine children aged four to six with ADHD. Two-thirds of the children were boys. Beauchaine believed that often these children had strained relationships with their peers, teachers, and parents. Thus, during the sessions, parents were taught better disciplining strategies. They were reminded of how they can sometimes overreact and get physical while trying to discipline their kids with ADHD. He suggested that it was common for parents to slip into negative behaviors when they felt frustrated and tired by the actions of their child.

He proposed that when parents were introduced to the concept of positive parenting, they instantly knew what it entailed. They knew that praises, smiling, flexibility, hugging, focusing on rewards and privileges, setting achievable goals and expectations can help discipline them in a less threatening and adverse way.

As weeks passed by and parents learned of effective problem-solving techniques, positive parenting responses, and adaptive emotional regulation, the children also began to depict improvement in their behavior. Additionally, following the intervention, it was also notable that the heart rates of the children with ADHD slowed down a little and their breathing became calmer. All of this happened in just two months when the researchers predicted that the behavioral changes would start to show well after one year. To further prove that the behavioral improvements were the result of the intervention program, he divided families into two groups. One group received 20 weeks' worth of sessions whereas the other received only 10 sessions. The behavioral changes in the first group were more evident and long-lasting than the ones depicted by the children of parents in the second group. In his concluding remarks, Beauchaine proposed that the earlier parents of children with ADHD started taking therapy and practicing positive parenting, the better the results will be.

How to Improve Misbehavior Without Yelling or Shouting

Parenting kids with ADHD is a challenge for many parents. It is a test of their patience and good judgment to the point where they end up making bad decisions while disciplining misbehavior. Yelling and shouting don't always work but choosing compassionate approaches surely does. Below are some friendly approaches to discipline misbehavior without losing your mind.

Keep it Short

When disciplining your child, be concise. Many parenting experts believe that the best way to discipline children with ADHD is to use fewer words. The more direct you are with your commands and orders, the more effective they will be. Be very clear about what is expected of them so that they can hear and remember it.

Don't Bully Into Submission

When we yell at our kids, we generate fear. This is no less than a form of bullying where they begin to behave out of fear not out of their own will. Thus, you have to show them that you care and look them in the eye when telling them how valuable they are and how grateful and proud you will be when they behave well. You can achieve a lot more when you talk to them, not at them.

Choose an Appropriate Time to Have a Talk

Every child wants to feel valued and respected. They want to feel validated and important. Thus, when they do something you don't like or agree with, ignore it instead of yelling at them at the moment. Choose another time to bring it up and talk about it in a calm and composed manner.

Be Proactive When Discussing Negative Consequences

Another great approach to handle misbehavior is to make them aware of the consequences that await them if they break the rules. When setting consequences, you can use strategies like time-outs or taking away privileges to discipline them and learn from their mistakes. If any other consequences put them off, communicate them beforehand to prevent misbehavior before it even begins.

Set Punishments for Misbehavior

Appropriate punishments are another approachable way as long as they aren't too harsh or demeaning. For instance, suppose the child has spilled some juice on the kitchen tiles. An appropriate punishment would be to ask them to clean the mess instead of belittling them for their poor handling of the glass and being hyperactive.

Notes:

Chapter 12: Honing in on My Child's Abilities

Before you can understand your child's strengths and weaknesses, you must first understand what normal behavior is for a child. It is true that all children are different, but there is a standard spectrum of age-appropriate behavior that all children should meet. While your child does not need to be at the very top of the scale, they should fall somewhere in the range in order to be considered as progressing normally.

Up until now, ADHD has been identified and responded to based on reactions to the symptoms that each child has. Now that we have a better understanding of what's involved, we can better come up with a course of treatment that will benefit both child and adult and help them to better navigate the ups and downs of the problem.

Executive Skills

A term you will need to become familiar with is that of executive skills. Most people will view this term in relation to being able to perform certain executive tasks like running a business or organizational skill. However, this is not the true meaning when it comes to ADHD. While the ability to plan, decide, and perform tasks is definitely a part of it, the focus should be on the word 'executive.' It is the ability to 'execute' those things you planned, decided upon, and want to do.

Every person needs executive skills in their daily lives whether they are conducting a business or not. Even the simplest of tasks require these types of skills. Think about a simple task you might ask your child to do, eating all their food on the plate. To you, it may be a pretty straightforward thing to do but to the child it involves…

1. Choosing the right utensil to use

2. Utilizing that utensil in the right way.

3. Deciding which item of food to put in the mouth first

4. Chewing the food

5. And returning to pick up another item of food.

In normal children, this is usually done without much fanfare, but the ADHD child may see something exciting in the shape of the food and rather than eating it may discover a number of ways to play with it instead. They may lose interest in chewing and swallowing and prefer to spit or throw the food offending others around them. Even if the child is able to function well at the dinner table, there are many other decisions that may affect his behavior. The relationship he has with his siblings, the number of other distractions in the room, and the risk-reward ratio all are part of the process.

A child without ADHD makes a normal progression towards adulthood with little or no problem, but the ADHD child may struggle with this process every step of the way. Every decision becomes a chore from what foods to eat to something as simple and normal as knowing how to comb their own hair and could present a potential minefield. The development of this skill is a gradual process, and it is reasonable to expect that a child will reach a relative semi-adult independence by the time they reach their late adolescent years. However, they will still need to be reminded occasionally as they progress towards adulthood at which point your primary parenting role will reach its end. None of this is possible for the child if he has not yet mastered these executive skills.

Of course, there are several different types of executive skills that a child must develop. These can be viewed from two different perspectives. First, we can look at them from the developmental angle, these are progressive in nature. In other words, the natural order in which children their age learn these skills. You can also view them from a fundamental perspective; in other words, in recognizing what they help the child to do.

Likely the easiest way to understand them is from the developmental perspective. Most people recognize and understand the abilities natural to a toddler, a kindergartener, or a primary school aged child. When you know the order in which certain skills are expected in each child, you can more easily identify if your child is falling low on the spectrum. Let's look at each of these skills and how they develop in the average child.

Response Inhibition: The ability to think before acting

Children who have mastered response inhibition are able to make the connection between stimulus from their environment and the associated rewards. In other words, they learn to respond to stimuli according to an expected result. It is a normal response to both humans and animals. However, those with ADHD struggle to maintain control over their actions and often react without thinking without regard to what the consequences are.

Young children are usually able to wait for a short amount of time without getting overly anxious or disruptive while older children are capable of hearing a decision from an authority figure without debating the issue or becoming argumentative.

Working Memory

This is the ability to recall information and connect it to present tasks. It involves bringing past experiences to mind and applying them to current situations. As a child gets older, they should be able to complete more and more complex tasks. A young child may be only able to complete a one or two step task using their working memory, but an older child should be capable of recalling instructions given to them by a number of different people.

Emotional Control

The ability to control emotions while working on certain tasks or waiting for expectations to be fulfilled is difficult for any child. Non-ADHD children usually master this skill and can handle disappointment at a very early age. Teenagers often have to handle all sorts of emotions as they navigate between test taking, heavy homework assignments, and a variety of stress-related incidents in their daily lives and can still manage to get their tasks done.

Sustained Attention Span

Normally progressive children have the capacity to not only pay attention but are also able to extend their attention span for progressively longer periods of time as they age without getting bored or distracted. Younger children should be able to do this for at least five minutes while teenagers should be able to hold their attention for at least one to two hours.

Task Initiation

Children have the ability to get started on a project within a reasonable amount of time without procrastinating. Younger children should be able to start as soon as instructions are given and teenagers should be able to choose a time to start without waiting until the very last minute.

Prioritizing/Creating a Plan of Action

The ability to create a step-by-step plan of action from start to finish on an assignment or a task. This skill also involves decision making in the process. The child must be able to choose which steps are more important and be able to prioritize them in proper order. Younger children should be able to find ways to resolve issues with their peers while teenagers should be able to develop bigger plans for choosing a university or applying for a job without minimal help.

Organization

The ability to create a system to keep their things in order early on. Young children, with a little coaching, should be able to figure out how to organize their room, school supplies, and playthings. Teenagers should be able to organize their things on their own without any coaching from parents or other adults.

Time Management

Time Management is the ability to determine the best way to make use of their time. It involves understanding how much time they have to accomplish a certain task and find ways to make the best use of it. To accomplish this, they must view time as important and something that should be respected. Younger children should be able to follow schedules and time limits set by adults, but older children and teenagers should be able to create their own schedules to manage the tasks they have to do.

Persistence

The ability to establish a specific goal and to stay on task until its completion without getting distracted or drawn into more appealing projects. Young children should be able to see small rewards as a powerful enough goal to persist in a project while teenagers should be able to work on a job for a day, a week or more to earn enough money to buy an object of interest.

Flexibility

The ability to adjust their schedules, expectations, and behaviors in the face of changes, obstacles, or other challenges in order to get their job done. Younger children should be able to adjust to changes and obstacles with little disappointment while teenagers should be expected to reasonably adjust their tasks when they are not able to get their first option without fuss.

Metacognition

Every child must be able to stand back and take an objective view of their situation and determine how best to handle it. This is a self-evaluating skill where they take the role of an outsider, mentally step outside of themselves and observe how they are problem-solving and make adjustments accordingly. Young children should be expected to adjust their behavior after receiving constructive input from an adult while teenagers should be able to analyze his or her own conduct in a situation and make the proper adjustments on their own.

Being able to understand these executive skills is paramount to understanding your child's developmental progress. These skills outline the very basic progress that every child should make and while it may not happen at the same time for each child, if your children's peers are steadily picking up these skills and your child is languishing behind the pack it is cause for concern.

Studies have shown that some of these skills happen as early as the first year of a child's life. For example, response inhibition, working memory, and emotional control seem to occur somewhere between the child's first six to twelve months of life. The planning stage develops soon after. You may not readily observe these skills as they develop but you see them when your child begins to communicate to you his needs and wants. He may not be able to speak yet but has learned to communicate, he develops strategies on how he will get you to understand he needs to be fed, he wants his blankie or if he needs changing.

In the second year, children develop other skills like flexibility, time management, and task initiation. They may appear as very simple forms at first but will become progressively more refined as the child ages. Once you recognize that your child is not keeping up with the other children his age you have a decision to make. ADHD comes in two different forms. Depending on which skills they are weak in the child is not able to either think correctly or your child is not able to behave correctly.

Notes:

Chapter 13: Educating Children with ADHD

Educating a child with special needs is a huge topic— worthy of many books— but today, we'll discuss the basics.

The most important aspect of special education. By far, it is clear that there is a problem and that the problem is defined. If a child goes to kindergarten without finding something seriously wrong, it's easy to assume that the problem is small. The problem is further complicated by the fact that many diagnoses of special needs are interrelated, or very similar in symptoms. (Sometimes, we actually know of at least one child who has been diagnosed with severe ADHD when it is true. The problem was close-sightedness; he walked about the classroom not because he could not focus, but because he was trying to get a better picture of the activities.) For example, ADHD is heavily related to dyslexia, dyscalculia, and several similar diseases, although it is not linked to the autism spectrum, although it has many more symptoms than any of the dysfunctions in common with mild autism. A kid who doesn't like to talk may be autistic or may have the syndrome of apraxia, or social anxiety, or a weak stutter. Or if you try to provoke a conversation, they may be deaf and unable to hear you. The argument is that, no matter how qualified, special educators cannot help a child if they use tools and techniques developed for the wrong illness.

Remedial education and education with special needs have some similarities, but they are two separate topics–as' special needs may include scholastic affective disabilities such as dyslexia, but they can include learning just as easily as beautifully. A good special needs system knows how to deal with talented children because talent is a specific need, as well as those who need corrective assistance. The identification of strengths must be part and parcel of the learning of every special child.

Indeed, a special designation for children who are' twice exceptional' and require accommodation is available in special education–' 2E.' A student who reads three degrees above their classroom but is also deeply affected by ADHD and needs constant attention to be at work–that's 2E. A boy who isn't psychologically dyscalculic, but who is also a musical prodigy who learns new songs within days–that's 2E. And most people understand these kids more often.

The same is true at home. If it is not obvious, these two fundamental principles apply equally to all the lessons that your baby teaches at home. When you refuse to recognize that your child is different from the others or if you believe that one thing is wrong without an expert assessment, you make a serious mistake. Similarly, learning that your child is suffering from dyslexia or ADHD doesn't necessitate treating them as smart as a' normal' child – they just have a problem they need to overcome.

Special education resources: The main, most detailed and applicable methods in the area of special education are: The Individualized Education Plan (IEP), the key elements of current, special education, and IEPs act as a recordkeeping, as an information source for potential teachers, as an instrument to measure the development of children. An IEP includes information on the condition of the child, documented behaviors of the child, and details of each method and resource used to teach the child. There is no individualization without an IEP–and therefore, no special education.

A child's doctor and/or education counselors will inform you whether they have been diagnosed with an IEP condition. Not all children with a diagnosis need special education. There are many ADHD children who have gone to mainstream school without an IEP, and there are certainly those who need a special effort, even if they get and use drugs such as Concerta and Adderall properly without IEP, they will still not perform. It is a part of the process to determine if a certain child can cope with the' as-is' school system or if it needs appropriate specialist training.

The special education crew and room. It can be quite difficult to deal with a special child in the house— imagine six, eight, or fifteen in a classroom setting! There is clearly no educator who can foresee how the children will communicate, no matter how expert. When the ADHD kid leaps in part through a task, because he decides it is more fun to rotate in a circle than to add, and when he rotates, he smacks the child with the oppositional defiant disorder in the back of his head, what happens?

Would she scream at the top of her lungs and frighten the autistic student for a bathroom accident? Would she hit the ADHD boy and let him wonder why he's on the ground unexpectedly and bleeding through the cheek from scratch? Or is she going to just walk up to her desk and break up the whole room into a wild melee?

That's why almost all special school classrooms feature a' safe room,' where children can retreat to when they know that they can't cope with padded walls and noise insulation. This is also why each special educator comes with an assistant squadron. Some of them are specialist therapists, such as speech pathologists or ergotist; others are' just' other educators who have been trained to deal with and maintain control over an occasional whole-class breakdown.

You can learn from these realities as a parent. Of course, you already personalize the treatment your child receives— but do you keep track of issues you have, solutions you are trying to find, and how well they succeed or fail? Can you see how useful this will be in a month or two? Do you have a' safe area' in which the child will escape when overwhelmed? Ask your child's teacher what tools they use and how you can incorporate similar strategies in your home. Special training must not end— and should not stop— merely because your child left the classroom.

Notes:

Chapter 14: Improving Social Skills in Children with ADHD

Having positive companion connections and fellowships is significant for all children. Shockingly, numerous children with consideration shortage hyperactivity issue (ADHD) experience considerable difficulties making and keeping companions and being acknowledged inside the bigger friend gathering. The hastiness, hyperactivity, and distractedness related with ADHD can unleash ruin on a youngster's endeavors to associate with others in positive manners.

Not being acknowledged by one's friend gathering, feeling disengaged, unique, unlikeable and alone—this is maybe the most difficult part of ADHD-related hindrances and these encounters convey enduring impacts. Positive associations with others are so significant. Despite the fact that children with ADHD urgently need to make companions and be preferred by the gathering, they regularly simply don't have the foggiest idea how. Fortunately, you can enable your youngster to build up these social aptitudes and skills.

Expanding Your Child's Social Awareness

Research sees that children with ADHD tend as very poor screens of their own social conduct. They regularly don't have an unmistakable comprehension or attention to social circumstances and the responses they incite in others. They may feel that a cooperation with a friend went well, for instance, when it plainly didn't. ADHD-related challenges can bring about shortcomings in this capacity to precisely survey or "read" a social circumstance, self-assess, self-screen, and modify as important. These aptitudes must be instructed legitimately to your kid.

Show Skills Directly and Practice, Practice, Practice

Children with ADHD will in general experience considerable difficulties gaining from past encounters. They regularly respond without thoroughly considering outcomes. One approach to help these children is to give quick and successive criticism about wrong conduct or social miscues. Pretending can be useful to instruct, model, and practice positive social aptitudes, just as approaches to react to testing circumstances like prodding.

Start by concentrating on a couple of zones your youngster is battling with the most. This guarantees the learning procedure doesn't turn out to be excessively overpowering.

Numerous children with ADHD experience issues with the nuts and bolts, such as beginning and keeping up a discussion or cooperating with someone else in an equal way (for instance, tuning in, getting some information about the other kid's thoughts or sentiments, alternating in the discussion, or indicating enthusiasm for the other youngster), arranging and settling clashes as they emerge, sharing, keeping up close to home space, and in any event, talking in an ordinary manner of speaking that isn't excessively uproarious.

Obviously distinguish and offer data to your kid about social standards and the practices you need to see. Practice these pro-social aptitudes over and over and once more. Shape positive practices with quick compensates.

Make Opportunities for Friendship Development

For preschool and primary school-age children, play dates give a great chance to guardians to mentor and demonstrate positive friend collaborations for their kid and for the kid to rehearse these new abilities. Set up these recesses between your youngster and each or two companions in turn—as opposed to a gathering of companions. Structure the recess with the goal that your youngster can be best.

Consider yourself your youngster's "companionship mentor." Carefully consider the time span a playdate will run and pick exercises that will keep your kid generally intrigued.

As a youngster gets more established, peer connections and companionships are regularly increasingly confounded, yet it is similarly significant for you to keep on being included and to encourage positive friend collaborations. The center school and secondary school years can be severe for a youngster who battles socially. Regardless of whether a kid stays unaccepted by the companion bunch everywhere, having in any event one great companion during these years can regularly shield the youngster from the all-out negative impacts of exclusion by the friend gathering.

Center or high children who have encountered social separation and rehashed dismissal may feel frantic to have a place with any friend bunch that acknowledges them—even one with a negative impact.

Research and engage in bunches in your locale that cultivate positive friend connections and social abilities improvement like Boy Scouts, Indian Guides, Girl Scouts, Girls on the Run, sports groups, and so on. Ensure the gathering chiefs or mentors know about ADHD and can make a strong and positive condition for learning pro-social aptitudes.

Speak with the school, mentors, and neighborhood guardians so you realize what is new with your kid and with whom your youngster is investing energy. A youngster's friend gathering and the qualities of this gathering impact the people inside the gathering.

Work with The School To Improve Peer Status

When a youngster is marked by their companion bunch in a negative path due to social ability shortfalls, it tends to be extremely difficult to dissipate this notoriety. Truth be told, having negative notoriety is maybe probably the biggest obstruction your kid may need to defeat socially.

Studies have discovered that the negative friend status of children with ADHD is frequently effectively settled by right on time to-center primary school years and this notoriety can stay with the youngster even as the person in question starts to roll out constructive improvements in social abilities. Thus, it very well may be useful for guardians to work with their kid's instructors, mentors, and so on to attempt to address these reputational impacts.

Set up a positive working association with your youngster's educator. Enlighten them concerning your kid's zones of solidarity and interests, just as what they've been battling with. Offer any systems you've discovered supportive when taking a shot at your youngster's regions of shortcoming.

Little youngsters frequently look to their instructors when shaping social inclinations about their friends. An educator's glow, tolerance, acknowledgment, and delicate redirection can fill in as a model for the friend gathering and have some impact on a kid's economic wellbeing.

At the point when a kid has encountered disappointments in the study hall, it turns out to be much increasingly more significant for the youngster's instructor to deliberately discover approaches to cause positive to notice that kid. One approach to do this is to dole out the youngster exceptional errands and obligations within the sight of different children in the study hall.

Ensure these are duties in which your youngster can encounter achievement and grow better sentiments of self-esteem and acknowledgment inside the homeroom. Doing this likewise gives chances to the friend gathering to see your kid in a positive light and may stop the gathering procedure of companion dismissal. Blending the kid up with a sympathetic "amigo" inside the study hall can likewise help encourage social acknowledgment.

Work together with your kid's instructor to ensure the study hall condition is as "ADHD-accommodating" as would be prudent so your youngster is better ready to oversee ADHD manifestations. Work together with the educator (and mentor or another grown-up parental figure) on powerful conduct the board draws near, just as social aptitudes preparing.

Drug, when fitting, is regularly useful in lessening the negative practices that friends find off-putting. In the event that your kid is taking drugs to help oversee side effects of ADHD, make certain to work intently and cooperatively with your kid's primary care physician. All together for the drug to give the ideal advantage that it can in dealing with the center ADHD side effects, there is frequently a continuous need to screen, calibrate, and make changes en route.

Notes:

Chapter 15: ADHD Friendly Gadgets, Applications, Devices

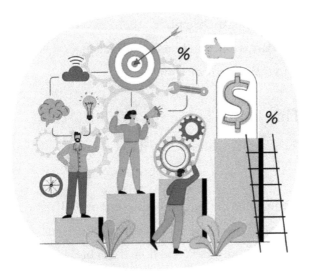

We're lucky to be growing and thriving in a world of technology that supports our ADHD, not one that shames us for the things we can't control. Though it can still be a daily struggle, managing our ADHD has never been easier will all the friendly technology, apps, and gadgets there are out there.

ADHD-Friendly Alarm Clocks

If you haven't already, you need to invest in an ADHD friendly alarm clock. One of the most popular kinds I've seen are those that actually have wheels, so you have to get up out of bed to turn them off! If you can't afford to buy one like this at the moment, simply moving your alarm clock across the room might help you get out of bed much easier in the morning rather than hitting the snooze over and over again.

There are even alarm clocks that will shoot things across the room that you have to put back in place. Alternatively, free apps on your phone like Alarms will go off and give challenges that you have to complete to make the noise stop!

How This Helps Someone With ADHD

Anyone who suffers from ADHD symptoms will know that irregular sleep is one of the big ones.

Whether you're having trouble getting out of bed because you are lost in a dream, or you're exhausted from a restless sleep and staying up all night due to distraction, it can be very challenging to listen to that first ring of the alarm clock. Using an ADHD friendly alarm clock will help you actually get out of bed and stay out.

There's no mind that can figure things out quite like an ADHD one, however. I've tried a few different alarm systems, but even my groggy mind can find a loophole in some that make it hard for me to get out of bed. Make sure to try your new alarm clock out on a night when you're not totally dependent on getting up at the crack of dawn.

Keyless Locks

Even those that don't struggle with ADHD might find that they are constantly losing their keys. Not only can this prevent you from getting inside, but it can also cause a great deal of stress.

Invest in keyless locks, ones you can open with technology or a code, in order to cut out the stress of losing keys! This will help those with ADHD because you won't have to worry about losing your keys anymore.

Weighted Blankets

Don't forget the important benefits of weighted blankets! One method of making your own is to invest in some scrap fabric and create a quilt. Before sewing it closed, add dry rice to areas at a time, sewing in lines of the rice in order to create a weighted effect. Beware- you cannot wash this homemade blanket! If you spill something on it, it might be toast, or else you're going to cook the rice that's inside!

This is still a good alternative if you're waiting for your weighted blanket in the mail or want to test out this method before committing to it.

Shower Clock

The shower is where I can come up with some of my greatest ideas, but it can also be the place for the most distraction! In order to help me stay on time in the shower, I would listen to music and know after two, three, or four songs (depending on length) that it was time to get out. This helped sometimes, but I would also realize after a few solos and using the shampoo bottle as a microphone in the shower that I was supposed to get out two songs ago. In order to stop this distraction once and for all, I put a shower clock in my tub so that I knew when 10- or 15-minutes had hit so I could actually get out on time.

Don't just use these clocks for the shower, either. Put one in the kitchen when you might be chopping things slowly, or in the living room when you're getting distracted watching TV. While you might think, "I have a clock on my phone," it's not one that's always there. If you can see that it's 1:00, then 1:01, then 1:02 on the clock on your wall, you know it's time to cut things short. You would probably only check the time every couple of minutes on your phone, making you lose chunks of time.

Fidget Toys

Those with ADHD might find that they simply cannot sit still with their hands empty. One great thing to keep around are different small toys, whether it's something that spins, clicks, or is covered in buttons to press.

When you can keep your hands busy, you keep your mind busy and out of trouble. If you look up "fidget toy" on any major site, you will be able to find a plethora of fun little distracting gadgets to choose from.

ADHD Apps

Luckily, we don't have to go to a physical store to get help for our ADHD, just the app store! Some of these are for your browser, other for your phone, and you might even need to pay for some. There are usually free trials or alternatives for most, but remember that a few extra dollars can go a long way if it means changing your life for the better.

Freedom

Freedom is an app that will actually block your computer from going online during certain time frames. This is wonderful for me, especially because I would find that I was done with work at 8 P.M. but would often spend my nights mindlessly scrolling the internet until midnight or later.

This will allow you to see when your internet time is going away so you can use it more efficiently.

ADHD Friendly Tech

Never stop looking for more ADHD friendly tech that you can include in your life. The smallest changes can have the biggest impacts, so do not underestimate the abilities of something you might have heard of that you did not originally think would help!

Alternative Clocks

We already mentioned shower clocks and different alarm clocks, but you should also think about investing in one that causes you to look at time in a completely different way.

Those that suffer from ADHD have time management issues because of distraction, but also simply sometimes because of the complexities that come along with trying to understand time.

An alternative clock, such as an hourglass, helps you to understand time in a more quantitative way rather than simply watching numbers change digitally. Other clocks might include actual sundials, or things that are similar in concept to hourglasses.

Smart Home Devices

There are so many devices out there that can turn an ordinary home into a place made for those with ADHD. One thing that I absolutely adore is the ability to check my stove, my locks, and that all doors have been closed. These are all done on different apps, but I used to have so many days where I would think, "Did I close the door? Did I turn off the oven?" and the distraction would ruin my workflow. I never forgot to do these things, yet I would always fear that I had. Apps let me check in on my home to make sure that I haven't missed anything, giving me the peace of mind I need to continue throughout my day.

Online Planners

On any smartphone, you have a calendar. However, it's better to get a different planner that will specifically help us ADHD sufferers. This way, you can plan what you're doing, how much work needs to be done, and plan for time for distractions, as well. Try out a few different calendars at once. You will eventually find one that you go to one more than others, meaning this is your best method! The more you can specify a calendar to your lifestyle, the easier it will be to eliminate distractions.

Notes:

Chapter 16: How Do You Speak to A Child With ADHD?

Communication using a child with ADHD gifts challenges for the parents. Most parents find it bothersome to receive their kid to slow down, listen and follow instructions. The issue is compounded if parents also have ADHD.

Communication Tips

Since it is crucial to communicate more efficiently with our kids, martin urges that teachers and parents try these plans.

- Provide clear, specific instructions.
- Attempt to split tasks into a couple of measures in order that they don't feel overwhelming.
- Give the child options.
- Ask questions rather than making announcements. This compels a young child to stop and consider the choices.

Life with a child or adolescent with attention deficit hyperactivity disorder (ADHD or add) may be bothersome, even overpowering. However, as a parent, you can help your child overcome daily struggles, channel their power in positive landscapes, and attract increased calm to your loved ones. Along with the sooner and more frequently you tackle your child's issues, the higher chance they need for succeeding in life.

Kids using ADHD normally have shortages in the executive role: the capacity to plan and think ahead, arrange, control impulses, and complete jobs. This usually means you have to take more than the executive, supplying extra advice while your kid slowly gets executive abilities of their very own.

Even though the symptoms of ADHD may be nothing short of exasperating, it is important not to forget that the kid who's dismissing, bothersome, or embarrassing you're not behaving. Children with ADHD wish to sit silently; they would like to produce their rooms clean and coordinated; they would like to do whatever their parent claims to perform --but they still do not understand how to create these things occur.

If you remember that having ADHD is equally as annoying to the child, it'll be a good deal simpler to react in positive, encouraging ways. With compassion, patience, and tons of assistance, you are able to handle youth ADHD when enjoying a secure, happy house.

ADHD along with your loved ones

Before you can successfully parent a child with ADHD, it is vital to know the effect of your child's symptoms in your household as a whole. Children with ADHD display a ton of behaviors that could disrupt family life. They frequently don't "hear" parental directions, so that they do not follow them. They are disorganized and easily diverted, maintaining other household members awaiting. Or they begin jobs and neglect to complete them let alone clean them up. Kids with impulsivity problems frequently interrupt discussions, need attention at improper times, and talk before they believe, stating tactless or embarrassing items. It is often tough to get them to bed and to sleep soundly. Hyperactive kids may rip around the home or even place themselves in bodily danger.

Due to these behaviors, siblings of kids with ADHD confront a number of challenges. Their demands often get much less attention than people of their kid with ADHD. They could possibly be rebuked more harshly if they vibrate, along with their successes, might be less renowned or taken for granted. They might be appreciated as helper parents blamed if the intruder with ADHD misbehaves under their oversight. Because of this, elephants might locate their love for a sister or brother with ADHD, combined with jealousy and bitterness.

The requirements of tracking your child with ADHD may be physically and emotionally exhausting. Your kid's inability to "listen" may result in frustration and frustration to anger followed by remorse about being mad at your son or daughter. Your kid's behavior can cause you to be nervous and worried. When there's a simple difference between your character and that of your kid with ADHD, their behavior can be particularly hard to accept.

To be able to satisfy the challenges of raising your child with ADHD, you have to be able to learn a combo of empathy along with consistency. Living in a house that offers both adore and construction is the very best thing for a kid or adolescent who's learning how to manage ADHD.

Notes:

Chapter 17: Homework and ADHD

One of the biggest hurdles in the life of a child with ADHD is homework. Sitting still and concentrating after a full day at school is very difficult. Everything, and I do mean everything, is a distraction from their assigned task. Many hours were spent by me yelling, threatening, and crying while my child sat distracted, frustrated, and emotionally out-of-control.

ADHD children are all different as are all children. Each has their own learning styles, energy levels, focusing abilities, ability to control their moods, frustration levels and stressors. You must find an approach that works best for your son or daughter.

1. When getting ready to do their homework your child should first find a quiet, non-distracting place to work away from the hustle and bustle of the household. The kitchen table is not the ideal work place.

2. Remove anything that will attract the child's attention such as: their Gameboy, magazines, books, toys, anything from the desktop not related to their homework, other children, pets and so forth from their reach or from the room.

3. Close the curtains or blinds and the door (leave cracked so you can peek in).

4. Although it may seem like a distraction to us, as parents, some ADHD children concentrate better

with some white noise. This can consist of low music played in the background, radio talk show on low, a book on tape, or even just the hum of a fan. Ask your child if the noise is disturbing them. Younger children usually will work well with just the hum of a fan or low soft music.

5. If they have several assignments or a rather long assignment set the timer so that they can take a break every 15 minutes for younger children and every 30 minutes to an hour for older children. They should engage in some type of physical activity to wear off pent up energy so that they can sit still and focus. This will prevent them from getting overtired and unfocused which can lead to frustration and emotional outbursts.

6. When an ADHD child brings home a large project or assignment it is very daunting. Sit down with them and make an outline of the task and work on the project step by step. Have your son or daughter focus only on one step at a time until the project is complete. This will avoid a sense of frustration and overwhelm and will make them feel successful at each juncture of the assignment.

7. Many ADHD children retain better while moving so have your student write out notes on note cards so that they can read them while moving about the room. This works especially well for items that must be memorized.

8. My sons can't sit still in a chair and will actually fall off. We recently purchased a café style table with the high table and chairs for this very reason. Now they can stand and eat if need be. If your child can't sit still let them stand at a high counter or podium and do their homework. This will use up some of that extra energy they always seem to have.

9. Remind your child to keep working when you see their mind wandering. (Observe them for a moment or two before saying anything to be sure they are drifting and not just thinking. If they are not fidgeting and looking around a lot and seem thoughtful, they may be thinking.)

10. Always have your child put his or her homework away as soon as they finish. This will avoid a lot of heartache over lost assignments and forgotten homework.

Notes:

Chapter 18: ADHD and Learning Deficiency

The range of co-morbidities of ADHD is varied and can be dependent to some degree on the resilience of the individual with ADHD and the levels of negativity they face in their environment. For instance, one child may react to habitual social exclusion with anger (external) while another child subjected to the same negative influences may respond by withdrawing and may experience depression (internal) negativity.

Children with ADHD will inevitably experience some level of learning difficulty, so let's take a closer visual look at some of these learning difficulties which by their very nature are disabling to the normal development of children who have them. Note the additional practical problems that can apply. Hopefully, this will provide an improved understanding of just how complex ADHD can be.

Towards a Spectrum of Learning & Communication Difficulties

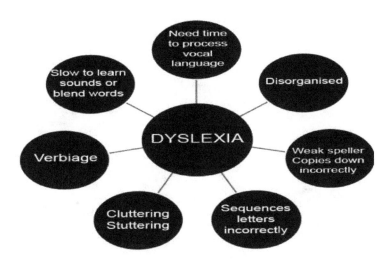

Reading & Writing Difficulties

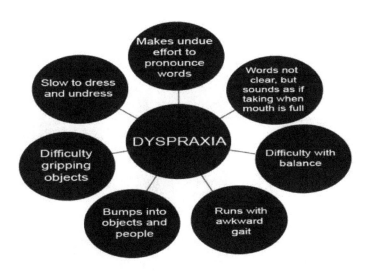

Physical Expression & Coordination

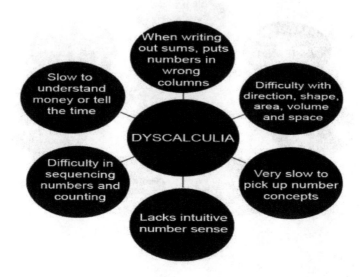

Numbers

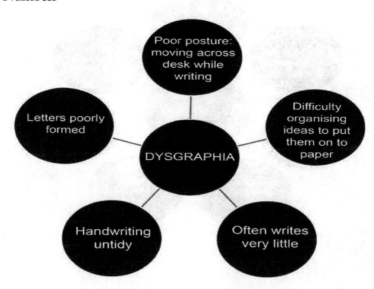

Letters

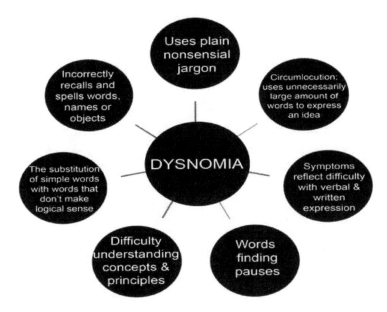

Take a simple task like asking a child with ADHD to complete a piece of homework for a subject they dislike or find difficult. Even with just one of the above-mentioned learning difficulties, the child will also possibly experience a fear of failure (atychiphobia), which in my opinion is a permeating symptom of ADHD.

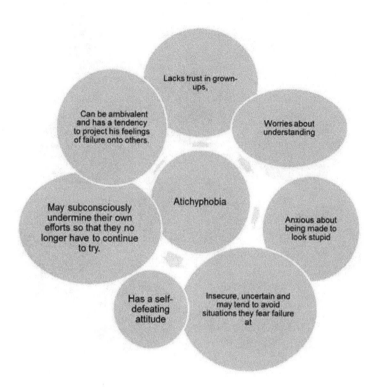

The child may experience frustration at the thought of having to concentrate, which will generate anxiety about the task itself, and the amount of time they are expected to take over it. This will often be expressed as anger, which will then accelerate their (emotional and possibly physical) hyperactivity. What goes up must come down, so this heightened state eventually descends into a low mood which may be permeated by feelings of shame, guilt, and embarrassment. This cycle can create a depressing mood of a fear of failure.

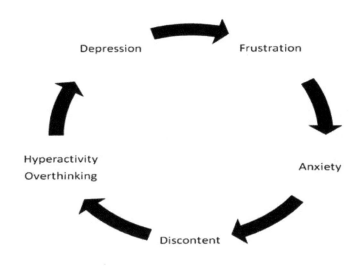

Cycle of Negativity

A major challenge to improve support for children with ADHD is to establish an accurate and full diagnosis for each individual, given that confusion often frustrates attempts to differentiate ADHD and other conditions when there is a high rate of co-morbidity between them.

It is also quite difficult to assess teenagers, as some of their symptoms can apply to the processes of normal pubescent development. This can make it difficult to determine which behaviors might suggest a disability as symptoms like irritability, disorganization and mood swings are a common part of adolescence. However, if symptoms are reported to occur to such a degree that they impair functioning, this may indicate more than just the stress of being a 'teenager'.

On the subject of age progression, some people think that people with ADHD find it easier to cope as they get older. My view is that as they get older people with ADHD can find it even harder to cope.

Society is less accepting of different behaviors and people with ADHD do try their hardest to conform and be accepted. In doing so, they suppress or disguise a lot of their natural presentations. This unfortunately places them under additional stress. Eventually they will reach their breaking point, and this can result in depression, social anxiety, and in some cases, agoraphobia.

As one moves through the transitional stages of life, there are increasing expectations from others. Also, remember that ADHD presentations are erratic in nature, so one can never predict how one is going to feel, behave, or react on a given day to a particular set of circumstances. Added to this is the fact that people with ADHD tend to act and feel much younger than their chronological age… and the frustrations of fitting in are often overwhelmed by the never-ending all-consuming fear of failure. Thus, societal milestones may not be achieved on time due to the child being too immature or not having learned the appropriate behaviors for their chronological age. This can generate anxiety that is often consoled with addictions like alcohol, tobacco, cannabis, gambling and sex.

It is of course, essential to recognize that levels of these ADHD and ancillary symptoms will vary from child to child, and one must not assume that one child has the same generalized symptoms as all the others.

It is also important to identify and understand the differences between ADHD and ADD (ADHD inattentive type) as the presentations are very unalike. Often where there is a dual diagnosis, support tends to focus on addressing the ADHD behaviors because these are socially unacceptable. Consequently, the other condition is often overlooked and the emotional impact of this can be developmentally detrimental.

Here are some of the different characteristics displayed by two children with ADHD:

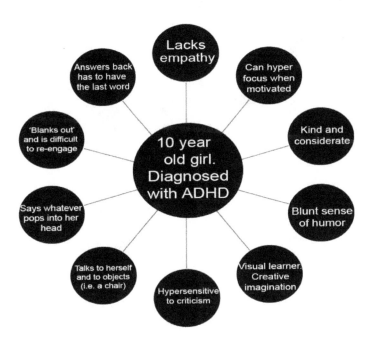

Child 1

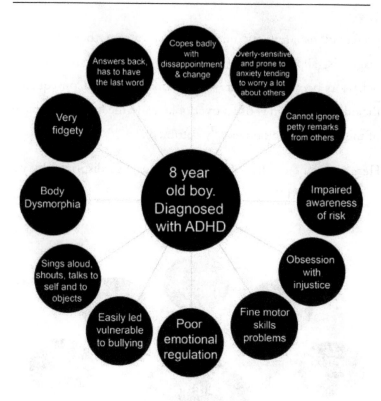

Child 2

Notes:

Chapter 19:   The Positive Side of ADHD

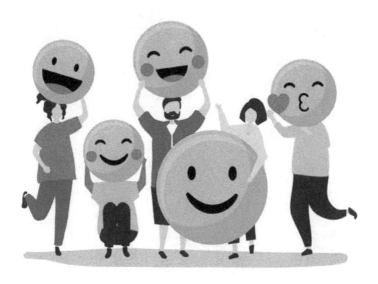

The first step in examining the positive side of ADHD is to transform your perspective. Stop looking at it from a negative viewpoint. Stop dwelling on the bad side of the behavioral issues, and start looking at them as beneficial personality attributes. For each negative behavioral trait, there is an opposite—a "mirror" trait that ignores the negativity and focuses solely on the positive. Below is a list of some of the negative ADHD attributes and their corresponding "mirror" traits. As you can see, it is all about perspective and how you choose to view each behavior.

- Impulsive behavior – Creative energy

- Moody and irritable – Sensitive and compassionate

- Easily distracted – Curious about the world around them

- Restless and hyperactive – Energetic and ready for adventure

- Stubborn – Determined

- Pushy and forward – Enthusiastic and assertive

When you focus on the "mirror" qualities of your child's behavior, you discover an entirely new way of living. You no longer have to cope with disruptive behaviors. Instead, you and your ADHD child can find new avenues to explore by using his "mirror" traits. There will still be times when those negative behaviors rear their ugly heads. But now you have the knowledge and skillset to deal with the negative behaviors swiftly, turning a potentially heated encounter into a positive situation.

In addition to finding the "mirror" qualities of your ADHD child, there are other positives to having ADHD. The ADHD mind might come across as unfocused and distractible, constantly leaping from one thought to another. However, this particular quality can come in quite handy for solving problems. As the mind of your ADHD child examines a problem with a peer, he is likely to sort through solutions faster than the non-ADHD child. While the non-ADHD child is still evaluating the first or second possible solution, your child has probably evaluated all of the solutions and may even be ready to solve the problem. ADHD children observe so many small details around them as they try to take in everything they see and hear. Your ADHD child probably hears much more than you realize. Just because your child appears to be involved in a different activity does not mean he is not also paying attention to your conversation. So, you may want to think twice before discussing adult matters in front of him.

Even though your ADHD child might have to work twice as hard as others, this is not necessarily a type of handicap. Instead, knowing that goals do not come as easily to him often intensifies the resolve of your ADHD child. His increased sense of determination pushes him to try and try again until he reaches his goal. Having this sort of determination may come across at times as stubbornness, but when you look at the "mirror" quality, you and your child will realize that persevering can be quite fulfilling. ADHD children are also not always unfocused. When they find an activity or task that excites them and keeps them intrigued, they can actually become intensely focused. This intense focus is so captivating that they often forget the entire world around them. Focusing like this can be quite helpful in completing projects, reading books, and overall learning.

Another positive side of ADHD is the seemingly endless amount of energy within your child. This type of infinite energy is useful in extracurricular activities, such as sports. Your ADHD child will probably want to participate in as many activities as possible. Baseball, football, and track are good examples of burning off that energy supply. While you may be concerned with injuries or worried that your child might fail, his thoughts are somewhere else. He is not as likely to be afraid of failure because learning to live with ADHD has taught him to persevere and push forward, no matter what. Even taking a family hike in the hills will be an adventure for your ADHD child. Not only does your child expend some extra energy, but he also gets the chance to spend time with his family. All of this physical activity not only keeps boredom at bay, but it is also good for your child's physical health.

Another encouraging aspect of ADHD is your child's ability to be compassionate and accepting of others. What someone might see as overly emotional is just your child being deeply in tune with his emotions and being unable to hold them inside. Sure, this can be trying at times, but in times of crisis, such as when a loved one passes away, you can almost bet that your ADHD child will be a great source of comfort. Compassion comes easily to your ADHD child. He understands and connects with emotions. In fact, ADHD children are often described as having the biggest hearts and sensitive souls. It is not uncommon to find your child crying during emotional movies because of his enhanced sense of compassion.

Your ADHD child is also likely to have a very accepting personality. It will not matter if a potential friend seems "different" than everyone else. This is because your ADHD child is already special himself, so he understands what the other child is feeling. Your ADHD child does not care if a peer is the "underdog." A friend is a friend, and your child will enjoy having a new companion to play with and share creative energy. ADHD children have big personalities to match their big hearts. They make friends easily because they have such an interest in the world and what is happening around them. They have a zest for life that draws others' attention to them like moths to a flame.

One very important "mirror" trait is creativity. Your ADHD child is full of thoughts and ideas that need an outlet. His imagination is running wild at all hours of the day and night. Help your child to harness that creativity in a constructive way. Give your child a sketchbook or notebook so that he has a place to write down his thoughts and ideas, a place to draw the images that never seem to stop playing in his mind. You never know—maybe he will become the next big inventor! At the very least, the two of you can have interesting conversations about his thoughts and ideas. It is also a good idea if you embrace your ADHD child's imagination. Go ahead, get on the floor and play with your child. Maybe it is with Legos, maybe it is with a race track, and maybe it is just the two of you pretending to be characters in a fantasy land. Let your child's wild imagination help you release the kid inside.

ADHD can be difficult to deal with every day. There is no doubt that the constant struggle to modify and cope with behaviors is hard on your ADHD child, as well as the rest of the family. However, keeping things in perspective—especially a positive perspective—will help make each day just a little bit easier. This positive outlook will also rub off onto your ADHD child, encouraging him to embrace his differences and live his very best life for the rest of his life.

Chapter 20: How to Debunk ADHD Myths

Despite the increased awareness, there are still professionals and parents who do not believe that ADHD is "real" and insist that it is all a myth that parents use to cover up bad parenting and misbehaving children or medical professionals and drug companies use to conjure up ways of making money.

As a mother of a child with ADHD, there were many times I wished the disorder did not exist and many times I thought I would pay any amount of money to make it go away! Reality is: ADHD is not a myth.

Skeptics ask, "Is ADHD a medical problem, or an educational problem, or an emotional problem or is it a behavioral problem?" The answer is, "Yes." ADHD is often all those problems!

ADHD can be a chronic, pervasive and severe disorder. Yet, there are those who reject the diagnosis preferring to have a child with "just" behavioral problems rather than accepting ADHD as a diagnosis in the DSM. After all, the DSM is to diagnosis mental disorders and because of the stigma surrounding mental illness no one wants their kid diagnosed as having a mental problem. Some don't want to "label" the child as ADHD but don't hesitate to call him a bully, a problem child or a failure. Other people do not acknowledge that the child has any problems and as one teacher told me, "The only 'deficit' your child has is you." Or the other teacher who told me I was the worst mother she had ever seen and there was no wonder my child had behavioral problems.

Some people argue that diagnosis is too subjective and unscientific. Skepticism about treatment for ADHD relates to what seems to be an ambiguous diagnosis. Then there are those individuals who believe ADHD is "just" a medical problem! Here are some myths about ADHD and facts.

Myth # 1 "Parents believe they have the only child with ADHD in the world."

Fact: Hardly. Conservative percentages indicate three to five percent of school-age children have ADHD - that is one child in every classroom. ADHD is the most commonly diagnosed and misunderstood childhood disorders.

Myth # 2 "There is nothing parents can do; children outgrow it."

Fact: A combination of parent training, medical intervention, education accommodations, and behavioral strategies can help the child succeed in school, salvage self-worth, and improve peer and interpersonal relations. ADHD is not outgrown but rather for most children with ADHD characteristics persist into adulthood.

Myth # 3 "It's the parents' fault."

Fact: Poor parenting does not create a child with ADHD. Chances are genetics did. Parents need to become experts on ADHD, learn how the characteristics affect their child and learn positive coping strategies and interventions. By understanding ADHD, parents are better advocates for their children.

Myth # 4 "Just boys have ADHD, not girls."

Fact: More boys are referred for evaluation than girls - they're usually more disruptive, break and damage things, get in trouble, and have trouble with appropriate social interactions and therefore drawing negative attention from adults. Parents and teachers tend to under-recognize girls with ADHD because girls with ADHD present symptoms differently than boys. Girls are more pleasant to be around than boys with ADHD. Girls are more likely to have the inattentive type of attention deficit and are more day dreamy and moody. Girls who have undiagnosed ADHD have: impaired cognitive ability resulting in poor academic achievement; low self-esteem; impaired social functioning; and are at increased risk for substance abuse and pregnancy.

Myth # 5 "Children with ADHD haven't been taught the difference between right and wrong."

Fact: Children with ADHD aren't morally deficit too. An untrained observer may misinterpret the child's impulsiveness, non-rule governed, and lack of immediate reflective thinking as if the child does not have a conscience. Children with ADHD are not bad kids who are little criminals who deserve to be punished. They are children who need to be provided accommodations and interventions to enhance their abilities to perform and complete tasks and follow rules.

Myth # 6 "Put him on medication and if he's ADHD it will solve the problem."

Fact: ADHD is not just a medical problem. Medication is not the first, last and only treatment for ADHD. Some kids do not respond to medication and that doesn't mean he doesn't have the disorder.

Myth # 7 "Teachers know how to deal with children with ADHD."

Fact: ADHD is not an educational major and certification for teachers. Educators, to effectively teach children with ADHD, need training, information and support. Some of the ways teachers can be informed about ADHD is take continuing education classes at teaching institutions offering courses on ADHD, attend professional training workshops, and attend in-services provided by local educational systems.

Myth # 8 "He can do the work, he just won't."

Fact: Kids with ADHD do not choose to be ADHD. It's not their fault and willful intention to have a deficit in paying attention, controlling activity and impulses.

Myth # 9 "Schools have special programs for children with ADHD."

Fact: There are no classes specifically designed for children with ADHD and it wouldn't be a good idea to put all children with ADHD in one classroom! Despite similarities among the children with the disorder; each individual child is different with different needs and must be dealt with individually. ADHD is a recognized disability and may require special education, related aids and services.

Myth # 10 "School systems don't have enough money to provide for services for every child with ADHD."

Fact: It is true, schools don't have enough money to provide services for every child with ADHD; however, not every child with ADHD requires special services and the cost of classroom accommodations is minimum compared to future costs of delinquency, drop out and unemployment - or prison.

Myth # 11 "Prognosis for children with ADHD is lousy."

Fact: Prognosis can be lousy but does not have to be. A multidisciplinary approach with the child, parents, medical and mental health professionals, educators, and other specialists working together for the success of the child with ADHD can improve the chance for achievement and positive adjustment.

Myth #12 "ADHD is way over identified and medicated."

Fact: More individuals are being appropriately identified with ADHD now than before. The good news is children are less likely to be misdiagnosed, mislabeled, and misplaced within the school system.

Myth # 13 "There is no real test for ADHD."

Fact: True, there is no litmus test; but there are guidelines for diagnosing the disorder. The disorder was officially recognized in 1987 by the American Psychiatric Association who established specified criteria used to diagnose attention deficit hyperactivity disorder in the Diagnostic Statistical Manual (DSM), the diagnostic bible for mental health professionals. Throughout the years the definition evolved to reflect increased understanding about the disorder.

Notes:

Chapter 21: Alternative Health & Complementary Medicine

More than 40% of all Americans use some form of complementary, alternative, or integrative medicine. While similar, each of these three (3) medical treatment types have a distinct meaning.

Complementary Medicine means using a non-mainstream medical approach in conjunction with conventional medicine, separating each into its own treatment. Alternative Medicine is when a non-mainstream medical approach is used in place or instead of a conventional approach. Integrative Medicine is combining a non-mainstream approach with conventional medicine to construct one unified treatment protocol.

Regardless of the exact approach, for our purposes, we will describe all three together under the term Alternative Medicine. To further understand this non-mainstream medical approach, it worthwhile to note that most alternative therapies have two (2) first, is the use of all-natural products like herbs (botanicals), vitamins, and minerals and are collectively marketed as dietary supplements. In the past several years interest in dietary supplements has increased dramatically. The most popular supplements in recent years include fish oil and other omega 3s, Ginkgo Biloba, and echinacea. A second hallmark of most alternative medicine methods is the focus on mind and body practices. Common mind and body alternative therapies include acupuncture, massage therapy, movement therapies (like Pilates), meditation, and relaxation therapies accomplished through a breathing exercise, muscle relaxation, or guided imagery.

While alternative therapies were once dismissed by licensed physicians in recent years, it has rapidly received more acceptance in conventional Western medicine and has become increasingly commonplace for treatment of a large number of health conditions.

A. Nutrition

Doctors have long recognized the association between good nutrition and good health. Nutrition is the science of foods and nutrients contained in food. Nutrients found in food are used by the body to support growth, provide energy, and maintain and support body tissue. Thus, the study of nutrition examines the relationship between diet and health, including the relationship between diet and disease. Examples of chronic health conditions commonly associated with nutrition include Cardiovascular Disease, Obesity, Type II Diabetes, Osteoporosis, and Hypertension.

B. National Institutes of Health Office of Dietary Supplements (ODS)

The National Institutes of Health Office of Dietary Supplements (ODS) is an office of the National Institutes of Health and provides users a searchable database containing bibliographic information about nutrition and health and disease. The database called the International Bibliographic Information on Dietary Supplements, or IBIDS for short can be accessed free of charge.

The IBIDS database is provided under a collaborative effort between the National Institutes of Health and the U.S. Department of Agriculture. Searching the database simply involves typing your search terms in the box and selecting "Search."

C. Biotechnology & Patents

Biotechnology is the application of technology to manufacture products that improve biological processes for the benefit of living organisms. In medicine, biotechnology is the basis for the development of pharmaceutical drugs, diagnostic and testing equipment, surgical implants, assisted living devices, and nearly every other tangible product that improves patient lives and outcomes.

A patent is a form of intellectual property. Intellectual property is distinct from tangible property and refers to creations of the mind. Just as physical property rights protect a person from encroachment on tangle items, intellectual property rights protect a person from the encroachment of creations of the mind. Intellectual property is generally divided into two categories, industrial property, and copyright. Most often, copyright applies to artistic works, like song lyrics, music scores, poems, novels, artistic paintings, photographs, and sculptures. Industrial property includes trademarks, industrial design, and patents and generally applies to physical items that are of utility for human use. Industrial property includes the ideas, thought, and the reason that form the basis of an invention and are commonly expressed in mathematical calculations, engineering design, and the manipulation and combination of chemical processes and properties.

Most biotechnological creations are protected by patents. Most often, intellectual property rights are asserted to prohibit another party from using creations of the mind in their own profit-making ventures. In addition to patents and copyright, two other common types of intellectual property are trademark and trade secrets. It is important to remember that intellectual property rights do not imply ownership, but rather the right to control the commercialization of the ideas or expression in question.

Patents can be an excellent source of information about not only patented drugs and medical devices but about disease and health conditions in general. Since patents are organized in a uniform and consistent manner, the introduction or background section can provide an excellent review of current scientific literature about the disease and also detailed discussions about various health care topics.

Since patent applications are filed as long as five years before patent approval, these filings can give the researcher a glimpse into the future of the treatment, and sometimes even cures for various diseases and health conditions.

While three types of patents can be granted, the two most common patents related to health care are Utility Patents and Design Patents. Utility patents protect inventions and discoveries of useful and new processes, machines, articles of manufacture, or "compositions of matter." As the name implies, design patents protect the drawings, charts, etc. that establish the shape and physical characteristics of an object to be manufactured. The third type of patent is the Plant Patent and is reserved for the discovery or invention of a new variety of "asexually" reproduced plant. Again, plant patents are uncommon in biotechnology.

D. Clinical Guidelines

As the name implies, a clinical guideline is a document that outlines the clinical management of a disease or health condition. In this regard, a clinical guideline can be viewed as a blueprint for the doctor and health care team to follow to diagnosis, manage, and treat specific health conditions in patients. Like any blueprint, however, the doctor must also incorporate her knowledge, experience, and best professional judgment and alter her application of a clinical guideline by taking into consideration the particular physical and emotional state of the patient, as well as the patients set of values and beliefs. Therefore, in practice, the use of clinical guidelines by physicians is just that, a guideline used in conjunction with several other considerations to determine patient care.

Clinical guidelines generally cover every aspect of patient care, from diagnosis to treatment and prognosis and continuing care. The clinical guideline will typically also outline the risks and benefits of a course of action, as well as cost-effectiveness.

An important societal objective of clinical guidelines is to standardize medical care, thereby allowing patients regardless of income or socioeconomic status to receive the same high-quality medical care.

E. Agency for Healthcare Research and Quality (AHRQ)

Clinical guidelines are generally collected and approved, and frequently written by a national health care agency. In the United States, the U.S. Agency for Healthcare Research and Quality (AHRQ) acts as the clearinghouse for clinical guidelines even though many are written by professional medical and doctor and associations. The AHRQ collection of guidelines which can be accessed at Searching clinical guidelines at AHRQ is easy as the site uses similar syntax as a normal web search. Thus, to find a guideline for treating a specific disease simply enter your term in the search box. Likewise, to search for guidelines for conditions containing multiple words or phrases, enclose your terms in quotation marks. Finally, Boolean searches can be performed using "and" or "or" between words and concepts of interest.

F. Drugs & Medications

Drugs are chemical substances that have a biological effect on humans and animals. Drugs are used by physicians to treat, cure, prevent, and even diagnose disease. Additionally, drugs can be used to enhance or improve mental or physical or well-being. Both prescription and over-the-counter drugs play several important roles in medicine. Drugs used to prevent disease are known as Prophylactic Drugs, drugs used to relieve symptoms are called Palliative Drugs and drugs used to cure disease are Therapeutic Drugs. Drugs for these purposes are also called medications or medicine, thus distinguishing them from drugs used for recreational or illicit purposes.

While all approved drugs have specific medicinal properties, most also have side effects. Side effects are secondary effects of medication that generally have no therapeutic value in the cure, treatment, or prevention of disease. Side effects can be both good and bad but are most often the latter. One major challenge drug manufacturer face is developing medications that maximize the therapeutic effects of a drug while minimizing side effects. When prescribing medications or recommending over-the-counter alternatives, doctors consider both the "good" and the "bad" when determining the best course of medicinal treatment for patients.

G. Prescription and Over-the-Counter Drugs and Medications

The best single resource to research drugs and medications is the Drug Information Portal administered by the National Institutes of Health (NIH). Unlike a standard web database, a portal is a site that functions as a point of access to multiple search engines or databases on the Internet.

Notes:

Conclusion

No matter if people believe in the prevalence of ADHD in our society or how accurately we can explain it and treat it, many of us live in hiding due to the stigma associated with being impaired. The purpose of this was to try to shed a better light on the effect ADHD has on the residents of its closed community and how far some of them have to go to reach the resemblance of a normal life.

The phenomenon of ADHD, or any mental disorder for that matter, is still a subject of much debate and blind spots, which begs the need for reformatory actions. People with ADHD aren't the only ones in the spectrum to suffer from scrutiny and/or the lack of acknowledgement of their issues. They are not a burden to society; in many scenarios, they are the ones that carry it.

We've given a lot of practical tips, scientific research, and a personal account. After all is said and done, only you can decide what the best method of treatment for your specific symptoms are. Whether you choose to medicate with multiple prescriptions, or you decide to only use exercise therapy, that is completely up to you.

There are a few more things that are important to remember for all ADHD patients. You should always keep a journal of your symptoms, mood, diet, and activities. Whether it's a daily journal log, or you simply write down the basic notes and numbers of the day, recording the small things that could influence your ADHD symptoms is important. It will give you the ability to reflect on the choices you've made to see if any might be causing symptoms to worsen.

Make sure that you are utilizing the free sources around you as well, which are present online and with friends. Talk to others about symptoms, and find someone close you can open up to. Find communities through the biggest social media pages, and don't be afraid to start your own forum, blog, or another way to voice your journey.

Another hugely important diet tip is drinking plenty of water. Water makes up 60% of your body's chemicals, and within that, your brain is made up of 80% water. Sources of dehydration like caffeine or alcohol cause impairment in your cognitive thinking and judgement. A rule of thumb is to make sure to drink half your weight in ounces daily, and also to lower the number of sugary drinks you consume.

Always keep in mind that this is a journey that will take time. Some moments you might feel like you've managed your ADHD, and other times, you might feel as if you haven't made any progress. Be mindful of the obstacles to get accurate results, and don't be hard on yourself for the days that might be more challenging. Don't compare yourself to others, and remember that focusing on what works best for you is the most important aspect of this entire journey.

I would like to thank you for taking the time to read this book. I hope you learned a lot from it and found value in it.

If you liked this book, I kindly ask you leave a review on the Amazon page dedicated to this text. If you are not satisfied or you have some particular suggestions to make, you can contact me directly at info@iltuomeglio.it

I will be happy to receive constructive criticism to improve this text and to grow as a person.

Good luck: I wish you the best..

Sofia